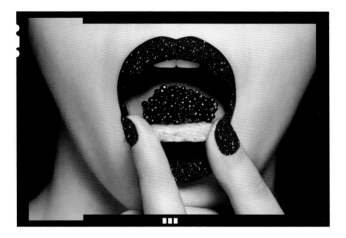

CHARLOTTE KNIGHT transformed her career path from nail technician to global beauty brand owner by following her passion for colour with endless determination. With a vision for beauty innovation and fearless determination, she rapidly became an industry leader.

Charlotte used her years of backstage and salon experience to develop the Ciaté brand in 2009. Charlotte's entrepreneurial spirit is an inspiration to those that surround her and her in-demand lifestyle resonates within each product within the Ciaté range. As Creative Director she ensures each product meets the needs of every woman's ever-demanding lifestyle – products must have instant impact, high pigment, luxe quality and be super covetable.

Knight has continued to drive the brand to success with groundbreaking designs and unique nail art offerings, and it is no wonder why she recently won Women: Inspiration & Enterprise's 'Ones to Watch' award for her leadership and innovation. The Caviar Manicure was a huge success for the brand, which Knight designed herself: 'I was working backstage at a shoot playing with different textures, glitters and effects when I tried pouring beads onto a wet nail and the whole set went crazy over it! So while doing a desk-side tour in New York I decided to wear this new manicure and the press could not believe the effect. The question on everyone's lips was "when can we get this?" The rest is history!'

Ciaté girls are pretty, fun and fearless. Unafraid to dream big and sparkle bright, they seek out shades and make-up solutions to explore fresh ways to update their look using fast, fabulous beauty solutions. Hotties on a mission, cuties with ambition – they are unafraid to express their own individuality and be their own kind of beautiful. These girls are made to make it and this shows in their make-up. They are their own muse, they make-up their own rules, when following their dreams they are unstoppable. With the mantra spread love, dare to play and live in colour Ciaté seek to make make-up empowering and above-all easy to achieve. Ciaté put the express in expression – from backstage to back-of-a-cab, only the cleverest application tricks, easy short-cuts and make-up hacks will do.

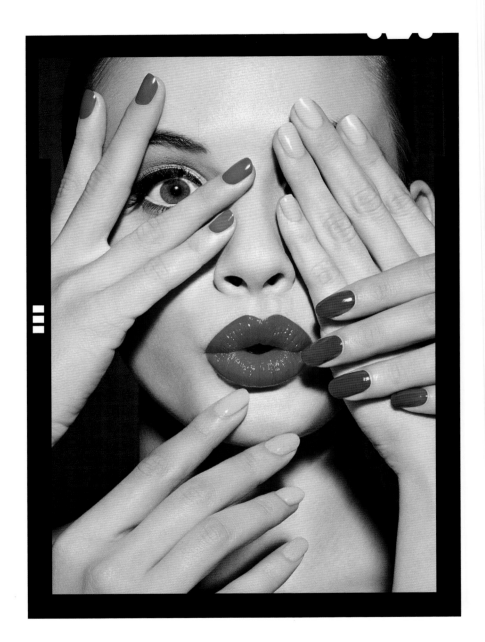

CIATÉ BOOK OF
NAIL STYLE

CHARLOTTE KNIGHT

PHOTOGRAPHY BY CLAIRE HARRISON

Kyle Books

For our fans, followers and fellow nail polish fanatics

First published in Great Britain in 2015 by
Kyle Books
an imprint of Kyle Cathie Limited
192–198 Vauxhall Bridge Road
London SW1V 1DX
general.enquiries@kylebooks.com
www.kylebooks.com

10 9 8 7 6 5 4 3 2 1

ISBN: 978 0 85783 331 0

A CIP catalogue record for this title is available from the British Library

Brand Agency Ltd is hereby identified as the author of this work in accordance with Section 77 of the Copyright, Designs and Patents Act 1988.

Text © Brand Agency Ltd 2015
Photographs © Claire Harrison 2015 except photo on page 23 © Karina Twiss
and pages 24–25 © Toby Lewis Thomas
Design © Kyle Books 2015

Editor: Vicky Orchard
Creative Direction: Charlotte Knight
Brand Direction: Hannah Griffiths and Sophie Huddy
Design: nicandlou.com
Photography: Claire Harrison
Manicurists: Rebecca Jade Wilson and Kimberley Nkosi
Illustration: Jack Slater
Production: Lisa Pinnell

Colour reproduction by F1 colour, London
Printed and bound in Slovenia by DZS Grafik d.o.o

CONTENTS

INTRODUCTION 6

THE BASICS 8

Basic Toolkit 10

Nail Art Tool Guide 12

Nail Care 14

Prepping Nails for Polish 16

Different Shaped Nails 18

Top Ten FAQs 20

Backstage Nail Tricks 24

Tips to Nurture Nails 26

Golden Rules For The Perfect Paint Job 28

How To Fix Any Manicure Problem 32

Top Ten Facts You Didn't Know About Nail Polish 34

THE STYLES 38

STYLE MENU 110

ACKNOWLEDGEMENTS 112

INTRODUCTION

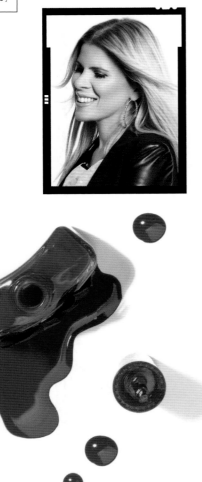

Starting out as a backstage session nail technician and now the owner of a global cosmetics brand, my journey within the beauty world has been filled with inspirational discoveries and sometimes incredibly awe-inspiring adventures!

Negative space, half moons and hoof sticks – the world of manicures is packed with its own tricks and terms and in this book you'll find an edit of every essential insider tip to make your manicure a whole lot more stylish.

For me, a manicure means so much more than polish – you'll find ways to care for nails from the inside-out and more importantly how to style them up to make a real lasting impression, after all – your nails really can be one of the most interesting accessories to any outfit, so make sure they make a statement!

The Styles section is packed with super pretty nail art looks along with step-by-step photos to help achieve each look. I worked closely with celebrity nail technician and Ciaté Global Nail Ambassador Rebecca Jade Wilson to create each look, making sure the styles ranged from simple and effective to high impact, high-end finishes, to suit all skill levels.

Charlotte x

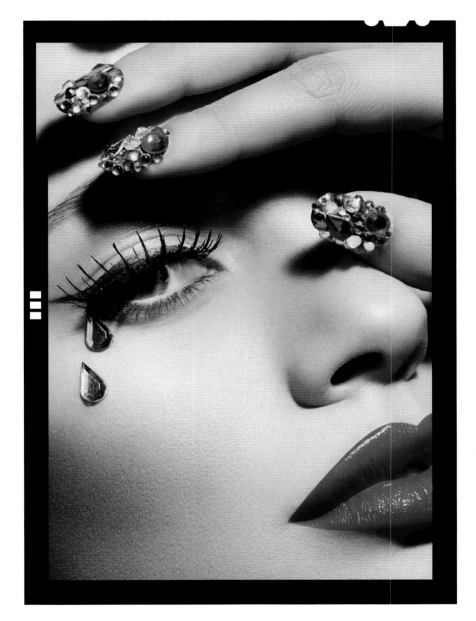

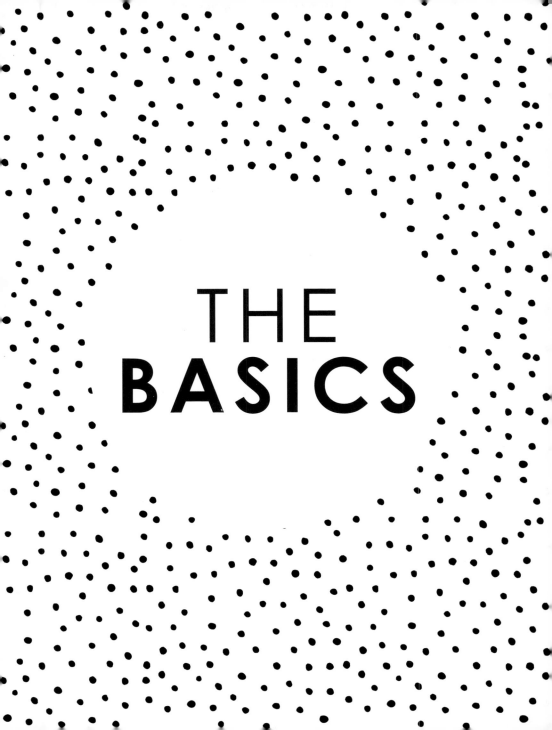

THE
BASICS

✣

BASIC TOOLKIT

• NAIL FILE

Ever since Marie Antoinette's 'lime à ongles' (a nail file-like tool made of pumice stone), shaped nails have become a grooming must-have and the nail file has been an essential tool in every girl's beauty regime. Here's a run-down of each type of nail file out there:

• emery board

The most cost-effective way to file nails is the classic emery board. Simple to use, they are practical and a beauty basic for many – however, they wear down quickly meaning regular replacements are needed. Brand new files can sometimes be too abrasive, rub their surfaces together to buff down the grit.

• crystal

Crystal files seal the keratin layers together at the edge of the nail, preventing peeling and chipping. They have the longest lifespan of any nail file and can be kept clean by simply washing with soapy water. They may be pricey, but are well worth the investment long-term.

• metal

Long-wearing and resilient, metal files can outlast the emery board – however, due to their tough nature, they are often better for working on thicker nails and can be too harsh on weak, thin or peeling nails.

• NAIL CLIPPERS

Ideal for snipping overgrown finger and toenails down to size, stainless steel nail clippers are simple to use and hardwearing. Be sure to trim from the outer corner of the nail to the centre to avoid painful ingrown nails.

• NAIL SCISSORS

Pick a small pair with comfortable grip handles and perfectly aligned fine blades for precision cutting and accurate trimming. Often the blades are curved to make nail trimming a breeze, giving nails a natural curved finish. They are also a nail art essential when trimming down appliqués, striping tape or embellishments fitted to the nail – flick to our Nail Art Tool Guide on page 12 to find out more.

• NAIL BUFFER

When you want to look polished without polish, this tool leaves naked nails shiny and groomed. Stick to buffing just once a month to avoid weakening nails. Flip to our Golden Rules on page 28 to read more tips on best practice when buffing. Avoid white buffer blocks – the strong grain will be too abrasive and will damage nails in the long-run.

• CUTICLE TRIMMER

Say goodbye to hangnails with this precision clipping gadget. The tilted blades help prevent over-clipping and allow you to swiftly trim away dry skin.

• ORANGE WOOD NAIL STICKS

Natural orange wood sticks are cost-effective and perfect for gently pushing back cuticles and cleaning under and around the nail without scratching the surface.

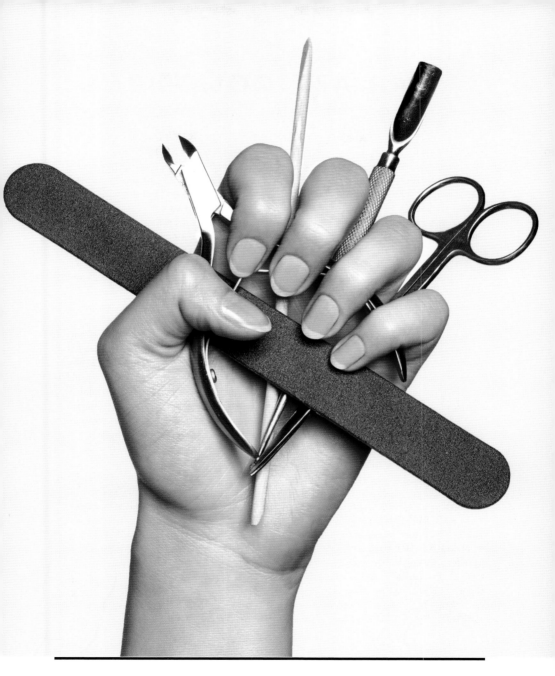

NAIL ART TOOL GUIDE

• DOTTING TOOLS

This metal tool is often double-ended and features circular ended tips. For perfectly placed spots of colour, a spotting tool is a must – available in an assortment of sizes depending on how detailed your dotted design needs to be.

• SHORT DETAILING BRUSH

This brush's bristles are short and stubby giving you full control of colour placement, for precision brushstrokes or skinny painted French tips.

• FAN BRUSH

This brush's bristles are fanned out into a curved shape – perfect for creating swirls of layered colour, giving a wash of pigment.

• FLAT BRUSH

This brush's bristles form a flat blade and come in an array of widths and lengths – great for applying clean parallel lines or one stroke of colour.

• STRIPING BRUSH

This brush's bristles are long and skinny, perfect for painting super skinny lines and negative space detailing.

• CLEAN-UP BRUSH

A skinny brush with a long tip; dip into acetone and sweep around the nail to remove any unwanted polish on the skin.

• STRIPING TAPE

This super skinny sticky-backed tape is sold in rolls and is available in a variety of colours from classic white to colourful metallics. Great to use as either a painting guide to peel away once polish is dry, or worn as a skinny line detail – ideal for cheating perfectly straight skinny lines if you don't have a steady hand.

• OMBRE SPONGE

Commonly sold as small white triangles of dense foam, sponges are the best way to dab layers of colour to the nail, creating dip-dye designs. Remember to pat thin layers of colour and build slowly for a precision finish.

• BRUSH CLEANSER

Acetone is essential in cleaning polish from brushes but can damage bristles over time due to its abrasive nature. Try not to soak brushes in acetone for extended periods to avoid this. Also, be sure to allow brushes to dry completely before using again.

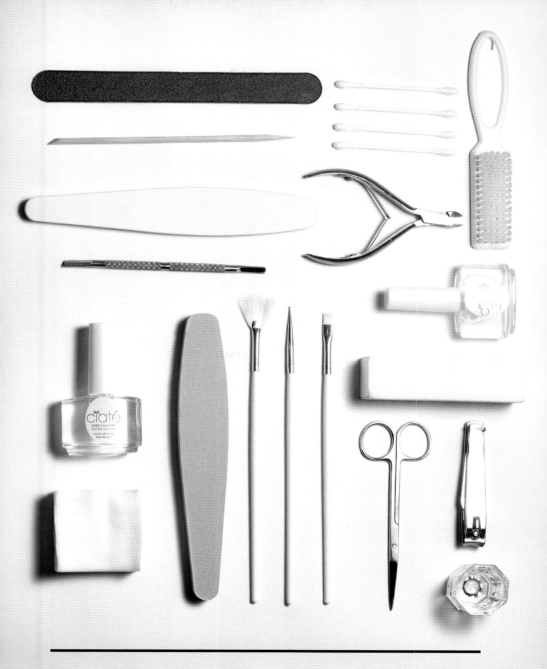

✳

NAIL CARE

WHO BETTER TO ASK FOR NAIL CARE ADVICE THAN A HAND
MODEL! OUR GORGEOUS HAND MODELS NOT ONLY WORK ON
NAIL POLISH CAMPAIGNS, BUT FOR A WHOLE HOST OF BRANDS
RANGING FROM JEWELLERY TO WASHING DETERGENT! WANT TO
KNOW HOW THEY KEEP THOSE HANDS PREPPED AND READY
FOR THEIR NEXT SHOOT? HERE'S HOW . . .

WHAT'S IN A HAND MODEL'S HANDBAG?

• I carry a mini bottle of almond oil with me and apply a few times a day to keep cuticles moist and minimise dryness and dehydration.

• A nail file is also an essential to save any snags and keep nails in shape.

• I also carry a cuticle pusher to keep nails clean and cuticle-free; I usually push them back after I've added a drop of almond oil.

WHAT'S YOUR BEST TIP FOR HEALTHY HANDS AND NAILS?

• My biggest piece of advice would be to invest in good nail products to keep nails in great condition – avoid cheap nail polishes and care products; you'll see better long-term results by using quality products.

WHAT NAIL RULES DO YOU LIVE BY?

• I don't have many nail colours, just clear high shine or matte top coats with ultra-conditioning ingredients.

• I do have a double-sided buffer which I try not to use too often to avoid thinning as it seems to increase nail ridging over time if I use it too much.

• I religiously use almond oil cream at night-time and add almond oil to cuticles – some people wear cotton gloves to lock in the moisture (I just can't sleep in them!)

• I keep my nails in shape by filing regularly on the go – I try not to grow them too long to avoid snags and breakages.

• I don't have any specific dietary tips but I like to drink plenty of milk as it seems to keep my nail tips extra white.

• I like to give nails a break from nail polish every now and then to avoid dehydrating them too much.

TOP TIP

I like to give nails a break from nail polish to avoid dehydrating them too much.

PREPPING NAILS FOR POLISH

TAKE TIME OUT FROM A BUSY SCHEDULE TO PREP AND PAMPER
NAILS BEFORE YOU PAINT – BY CREATING A FLAWLESS BASE,
YOUR POLISH IS MORE LIKELY TO LAST LONGER AND LOOK LIKE
YOU'VE JUST STEPPED OUT OF THE SALON!

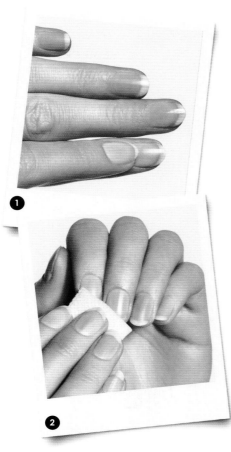

STEP BY STEP

1. SOAK OR DON'T SOAK?
Often the first step is to soak nails in warm
water making cuticle pushing easy, although
this is not the best start for your nails as
they absorb the water and slightly expand
– because of this, waterless manicures are
growing in popularity as a super dry nail is
more likely to grip colour for longer.

2. STRIP AWAY POLISH
Wipe down nails with oil-free polish
remover to clean away old colour or
treatments. Glitter polishes can be stubborn
to remove, so soak cotton pads in acetone
and wrap each nail tip allowing it to soak for
about 5 minutes.

TOP TIP
*Remember to
rehydrate nails
after using
acetone*

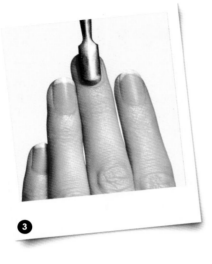

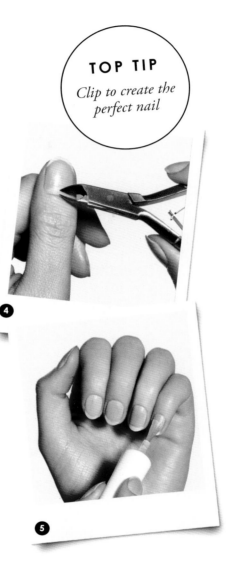

TOP TIP

*Clip to create the
perfect nail*

3. CUTICLE MAINTENANCE

Pick up a cuticle remover to make removing
cuticles extra easy – add a drop of cuticle
remover to each nail and allow to soak for
a minute or so, gently push back each
cuticle to remove excess and thoroughly
wash hands afterwards.

4. SHAPE UP

Use a file or clippers to create the perfect nail
size and shape – flip to our nail shape guide
(pages 18–19) for more inspiration!

5. CLEAN AND
CLEAN AGAIN

Use another sweep of nail polish remover
or a nail toner to remove any oil or residue
from the nail for an extra clean base to
ensure maximum colour grip.

DIFFERENT SHAPED NAILS

THIS SIMPLE GUIDE TO THE MOST POPULAR NAIL SHAPES WILL
HELP YOU TO CHOOSE THE PERFECT SHAPE FOR YOUR NAILS
AND HOW TO ACHIEVE THEM.

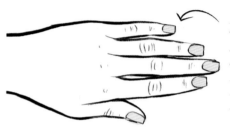

SQUARE

This timeless shape is a popular choice for a clean-looking, sturdy finish. The free edge of the nail is filed or clipped straight, giving it slightly sharpened corners. The square is ideal for a larger nail bed as it can sometimes make smaller nails look shorter and wider.

OVAL

This tapered nail shape is delicate, feminine and flattering, giving nails a classically groomed finish. Rounded from the tip all the way to the nail edge, nail edges are softened by gentle filing making them slightly weaker. Be sure to file each side of the nail evenly to ensure they look neat and symmetrical.

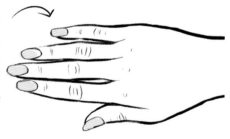

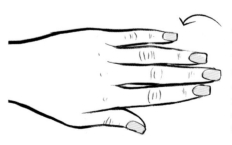

SQUOVAL

Combining the elegance of the Oval with the strength of the Square, the Squoval is a fashionable nail shape and flattering for almost all fingertips. It is also the best choice for strength and versatility – nail edges are straight, with softened corners to prevent snagging and scratching.

ROUND

Short nails are most suited to this natural, conservative shape. The free edge of the nail is rounded to follow the natural curve of the nail bed.

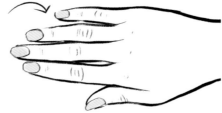

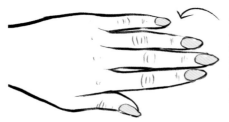

ALMOND

A recurring favourite of fashionistas, this long, tapered shape is super flattering, adding length to fingers making them look long and slender. Due to its excessively extended, curved contours this shape usually works best with gel or acrylic nails.

BALLERINA

Like almond nails, Ballerina nails are tapered at the edges, but end in a flattened point. Other names for this shape include Squareletto or even Coffin nails, but the flat-tipped, long point lends itself to a beautifully ballerina 'en pointe'. This longer length works best on gel or acrylic nails.

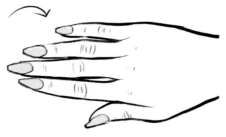

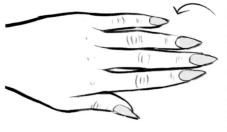

STILETTO

Just like Stiletto heels, this sharply tapered nail shape is a spiky point and seriously sexy. The stiletto shape is the weakest of all shapes and depending upon how sharp it is can scratch and snag. It is a fun shape and can be really flattering, especially for longer nails, but should be reinforced with gel or acrylic to avoid breakage.

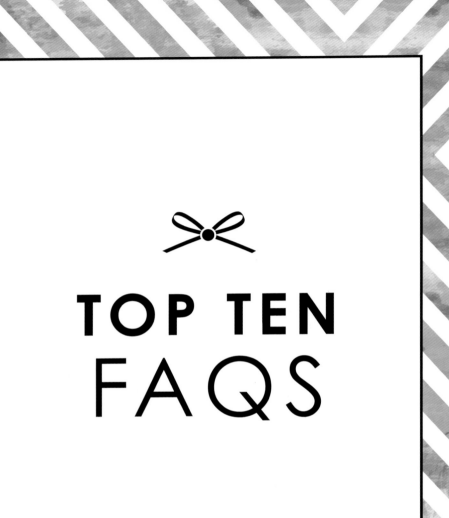

TOP TEN
FAQS

1
HOW DO I STOP MY NAILS FROM BREAKING?

The nail is made up of multiple miniscule layers – making them prone to weakness and the dreaded breakages. To stop nails breaking you need to get to the root of the problem – literally – by regularly rubbing cuticle oil to the base of the nail, which will encourage them to grow noticeably stronger and healthier. The cuticles are the root of your nail – if you want healthy and long nails you need to nurture them. This is a long-term fix – for short term results, use a strengthening treatment or you could consider a gel manicure which gives nails instant strength while allowing the natural nail to grow underneath.

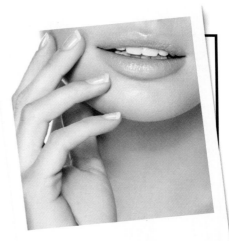

2
WHAT IS CUTICLE OIL USED FOR?

Cuticle oil gives instant, intense moisture to the skin around your nail which can have a tendency to harden and split. It is also packed with nourishing ingredients that seep into the surrounding nail and, over time, will encourage nails to grow back smoother and healthier. If you need a treat on-the-go, grab a cuticle oil pen, perfect for travelling hands.

3
HOW DO I MAKE MY MANICURE LAST?

It's all in the application – invest time in painting a base coat, multiple thin coats of colour and a long-wear top coat for maximum wear time. You should also consider how regularly you use your hands – when in and out of water or hard at work it's much harder to maintain manis – so consider acrylic or gel nails to give a longer lasting finish. The Ciaté Geltox Starter Kit allows you to transform any nail colour into a long-wearing gel finish, well worth the investment.

4
HOW DO I STOP MY NAIL POLISH FROM PEELING?

Nail polish peeling is a nuisance that can be avoided by using a good base coat and avoiding a heavy polish application. Nail health also impacts the wearability of polish, so be sure to treat weak and splitting nails to give your polish better wearing results and consider adding extra protein and B vitamins into your diet to ensure you are nourished inside and out.

5
IS NAIL POLISH REMOVER BAD FOR YOUR NAILS?

Nail polish remover is perfectly fine to use on nails on a regular basis – when using an acetone-free formula. Acetone is a solvent and has a dehydrating effect on skin and nails, which can sometimes be instantly visible as it leaves skin and nails white due to its oil-stripping properties. Many brands offer non-acetone formula polish removers which encourage hydration.

6
IS NAIL VARNISH REMOVER SAFE DURING PREGNANCY?

It is perfectly safe to use nail polish remover while pregnant, however, using nail polish regularly may be harmful due to high levels of chemicals including formaldehyde and toluene – so stick to free-from nail polish brands to avoid exposure.

7
HOW DO I MAKE MY NAILS GROW FASTER?

It's really down to nutrition and your body's natural keratin levels – each individual is different, some people's nails grow faster than others in the same way hair does. Give nails a helping hand by using nail treatments to add strength to the nail plate allowing your nails to grow with minimal breakage. Eating nutrient rich food is also essential (see page 26).

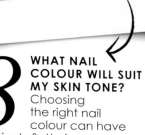

9 HOW DO I STOP MY NAILS FROM SPLITTING?

The delicate layers that make up nails can be weakened by water, humidity, wear and tear and overall nail health. Try to regularly treat them with nutrient-rich products to hydrate them – it may be worth taking a nail polish detox break and going polish-free for a few days to allow nails to breathe and revive themselves. Always use a glass nail file when shaping nails, as it will seal the free edge of the nail and minimise splitting.

8 WHAT NAIL COLOUR WILL SUIT MY SKIN TONE?

Choosing the right nail colour can have amazingly flattering, or sometimes unflattering, effects on your hands and skin tone. Fair skin with a red undertone works best with cool-toned shades, while yellow undertones suit warmer skin. Medium skin tones can pull off pretty much any shade, with creamy peach tones working best. Olive and dark skin tones are the luckiest of all and can carry off practically any rainbow shade you wish! But remember, beauty is about having fun, so embrace those out-of-the-box seasonal shades to add a pop of colour to your look, no matter what the rules are!

10 ARE GEL NAILS BAD FOR YOUR NAILS?

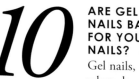

Gel nails, when done properly, can strengthen nails and encourage them to grow, while giving you the benefits of chip-free long-lasting colour. However, when worn back-to-back the nail can become thinner and dehydrated so try to take a break. Removing gel nails must be done correctly to ensure no damage is done to the nail plate; the heavy use of acetone and sometimes even tools to scrape away gel can damage the nail.

BACKSTAGE NAIL TRICKS

WHEN PLANNING AHEAD FOR A SPECIAL EVENT
MIMIC THE SESSION NAIL TECHS AND PREP YOUR
NAIL ART A DAY OR TWO AHEAD.

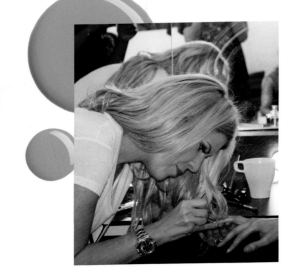

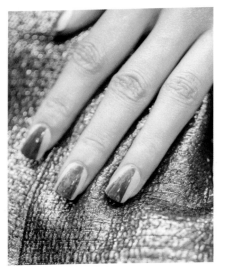

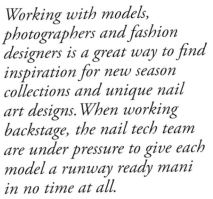

Working with models, photographers and fashion designers is a great way to find inspiration for new season collections and unique nail art designs. When working backstage, the nail tech team are under pressure to give each model a runway ready mani in no time at all.

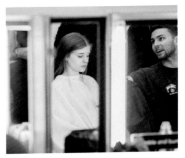

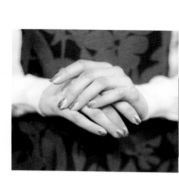

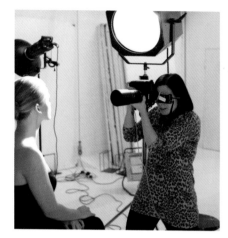

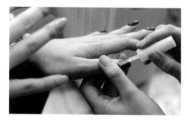

Often nail art designs are painted on false nails ahead of the show. That way there is no need to worry about smudging polish and models can get dressed straight away. Mimic this trick when prepping for a big event so you won't need to rush your nail art design.

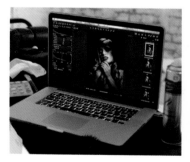

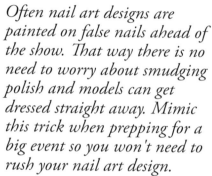

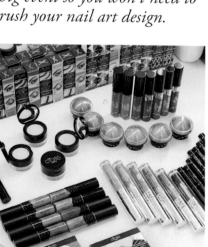

TIPS TO NURTURE NAILS

NO DOUBT CUTICLE OILS AND STRENGTHENING TREATMENTS
HELP, BUT YOUR DIET CAN ALSO GIVE YOUR NAILS AN EXTRA
HEALTH BOOST. HERE'S WHAT I LIKE TO SNACK ON.

Bananas, beans, cauliflower, eggs, lentils, peanuts, salmon
– for biotin (a.k.a. vitamin H)
Biotin is essential for your body to develop healthy nails (and hair too) – a deficiency in biotin may result in brittle hair and nails, so be sure to keep your levels topped up. A deficiency of vitamin B12 can lead to excessive nail dryness, overly curved nail ends and ridging.

Eggs, flaxseed, fish oil, mackerel, spinach, tuna, walnuts
– for omega-3 fatty acids
The three active ingredients – alpha-linolenic acid, eicosapentaenoic acid and docosahexaenoic acid – are all essential fatty acids and essential to the outermost layer of the epidermis that contains keratin, key for nail growth.

Chicken, eggs, lean red meats, low-fat dairy, nuts, seafood, soybeans – for protein
Nails are made up of structural proteins, most commonly known as keratin, making them essential for growing strong nails. You can find protein not only in meat but nuts and dairy too. A lack of protein may show up on nails as white bands or even the absence of the 'half moons' on nails.

Apricots, broccoli, egg yolks, mangoes, oatmeal, spinach
– for vitamin A
Vitamin A helps produce a conditioning substance for the scalp known as sebum, which keeps hair looking and feeling healthy. In addition to these beauty benefits, this vitamin contributes to better eye health and immune system function, which keeps you healthy and strong from head to toe.

Meats, eggs, wholewheat bread or pasta, kale – for iron
Iron is essential for healthy nails, skin tone and hair growth. If your nails are thin, curved or have ridges, it's usually a tell-tale sign of anaemia or an iron deficiency.

Green beans, pumpkin seeds, lean beef, lobster, oysters, soybeans
– for zinc
Zinc actively helps the immune system function properly, assisting the body's ability to build new proteins, essential for strong nails. A lack of zinc in your diet may be the reason your nails are weak or not growing, and may also cause white spots on the nail.

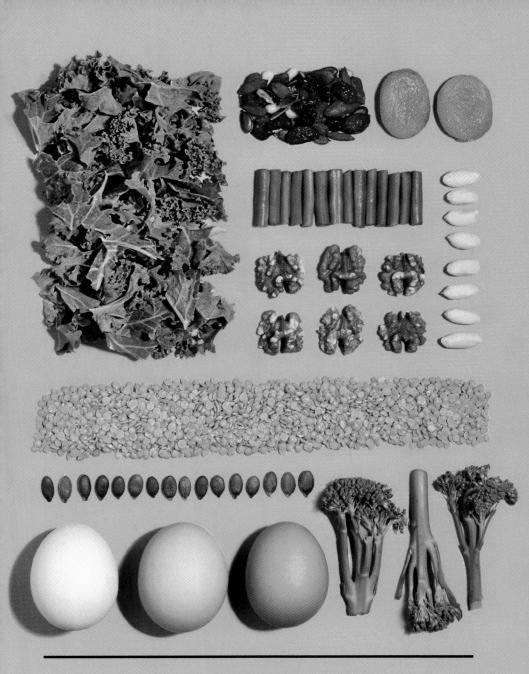

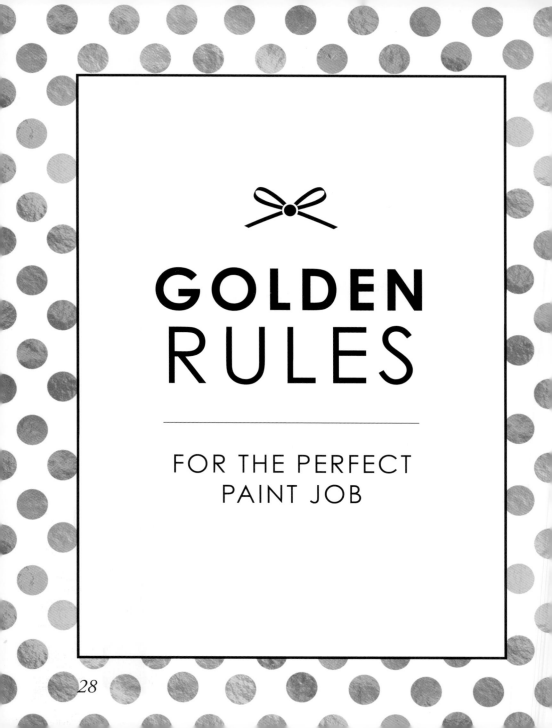

GOLDEN
RULES

FOR THE PERFECT
PAINT JOB

1 Nails must be completely clean before you begin to paint. Remove all traces of polish and oils using acetone or nail polish remover, which will strip colour in no time (even glitter shades)! Although try not to over-use acetone as it will dehydrate the nail and skin. Never be tempted to pick or peel away polish from the nail, this will aggravate and even damage the surface of the nail.

2 Not wearing any polish already? It's still really essential that you clean your nails to ensure no grease or oils are on the surface of the nail before painting as it will act as a barrier and stop your polish sticking to the nail or can even cause polish to bubble, or easily chip. Clean nails by gently wiping them with nail polish remover.

3 If nails are too long, avoid clippers and use a file to bring them down to a better length – carefully file from the corner of the wall inwards, to avoid the dreaded ingrown nails or even infection.

4 Once you have the right length, shape up using a nail file (check out the different options in the Basic Toolkit on page 10 for my advice). Never saw nails back and forth as this will cause them to weaken. Instead, choose one direction and stick to sweeping movements from the outer edge to the centre of the nail.

29

5 Nail shape trends are forever changing seasonally – from oval to square to stiletto. Choose the shape that looks best on you – your nail shape can help to elongate hands and even improve the look of your whole hand. Flip to my nail shape guide on pages 18–19 to discover a menu of different shapes.

6 Dab cuticles with a cuticle remover to soften skin, allow to absorb and gently push back using a cuticle pusher or an orange wood nail stick – this makes nails look instantly neater and longer, and means you don't need to use cuticle clippers which can be tricky and sometimes cause nips or tears to the skin.

7 Nail buffers are perfect for removing ridges and adding a natural sheen but use with caution, too much buffing can wear down your nails. Try buffing in the direction of the nail growth (rather than horizontally) to add extra sheen while minimising damage. Stick to buffing once a month and follow up with a strengthening base coat treatment to help nails stay strong.

8 Never, ever skip base coat: it stops any staining, protects your nails from polish and acts as a grip for nail polish. It is also often enriched with nourishing ingredients that promote strength and improve nail condition.

9 Don't be tempted to rush application with thick layers. Apply polish in a few thin layers, allowing each coat to dry in between to give a smoother finish that will also dry quicker. Dunking nails in ice water will also speed up your drying time.

10 Reapply top coat to keep nails glossy and help polish last. Using quick-dry formulas such as Ciaté Speed Coat makes this easy on-the-go. This is a great way to extend a salon manicure too.

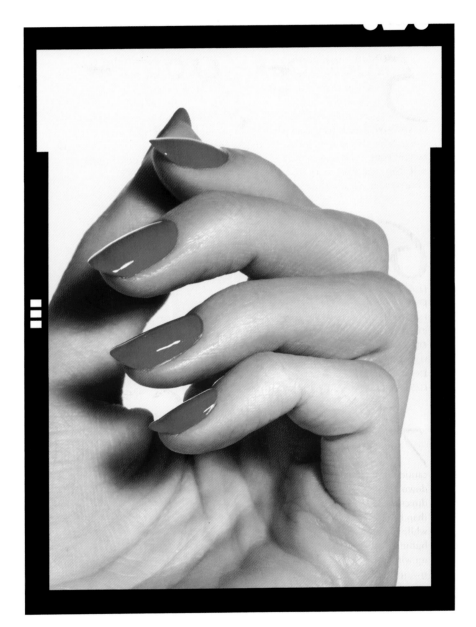

31

HOW TO FIX ANY
MANICURE PROBLEM

IF YOU ARE PRONE TO MANICURE MISTAKES, HERE'S A ROUND-
UP OF OUR QUICK FIXES FOR COMMON PROBLEMS.

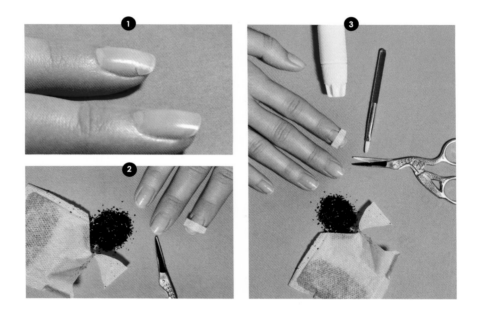

1. HAVE A CUPPA

Did you know you can fix nail splits using a teabag? Thanks to its strong mesh texture, a teabag is the perfect way to bind the nail and prevent the split from becoming a painful tear.

Cut the teabag mesh to size, lay over the split and paint a coat of nail glue to bond it to the nail. Simple!

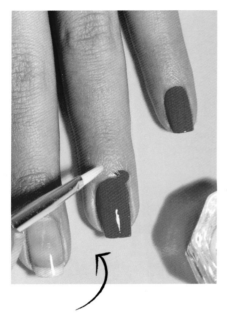

4. GLITTER GRADIENT

If you're suffering chipped polish and need to quickly transform them back to perfection, create a quick and simple ombre nail using a dense glitter polish. Dab to the tip of each nail, spreading upwards to the middle of the nail to conceal chips and create a glitter dipped tip.

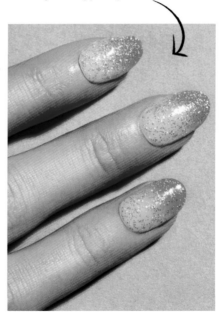

2. MESSY PAINT JOB

Tidy up any stray nail polish on the surrounding skin by dipping a skinny brush in acetone and wiping around the nail edge for a clean tidy finish. You could also use a nail corrector pen such as Ciaté's Perfect Paint Job.

3. STAINED MANI

Often deeply pigmented shades can leave nails and nail tips stained. Worry not! This can be fixed by lightly buffing the surface of the nail, or try soaking in baking soda to whisk away stains. To avoid this, always use a good base coat before you start painting.

5. CONCEAL SMUDGES

Fill in any dints, scratches and smudges by painting a layer of clear ridge-filling base coat to rescue your mani – the thicker formula will sit in the scratches to conceal them unlike a top coat.

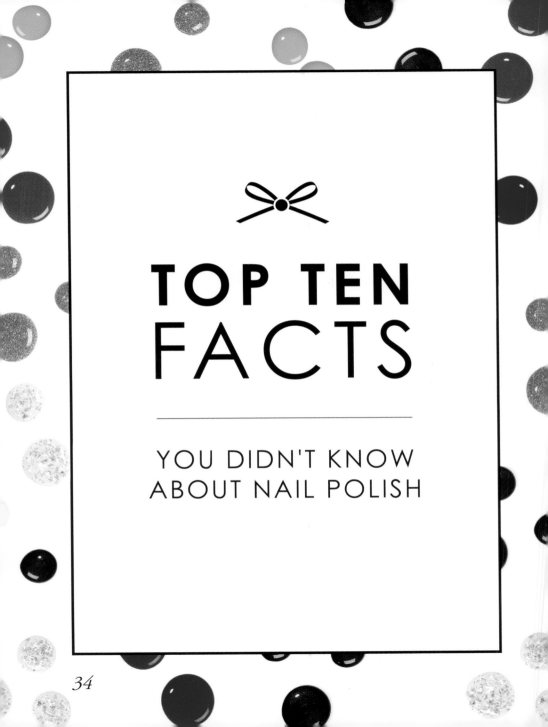

TOP TEN

FACTS

YOU DIDN'T KNOW
ABOUT NAIL POLISH

1 Your nail colour says more about you than you may think! Colour and human emotions are intrinsically linked, and studies have proven that your preferences are often a result of the relationship between unrelated items subconsciously stored in your memories. So next time you pick your paint shade, beware you may be giving away more than you think! For example, green is linked to confidence, orange to energy and red to power.

2 Back in the 1300s making your own nail polish was considered the norm. Beeswax, egg whites and vegetable dyes were some of the ingredients used by women to decorate nails – we'll never take polish for granted again!

3 The French manicure really did come from France. Members of French royalty distinguished themselves from the lower classes with groomed, elegant nail tips.

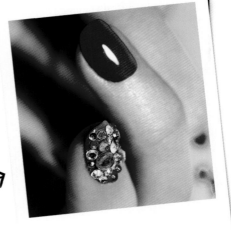

4 Nail polish started out as car paint. Revlon started making nail polish as we know it today in the 1920s using refined paint originally used to coat cars!

5 Did you know that nail polish remover never expires, meaning that the bottle in your cosmetics cupboard can last a lifetime…or even longer!

6 Sadly it's not the same story for nail polish. Once opened, a bottle of nail polish has a lifespan of approximately three years. Perfect excuse for an annual splurge on nail colour!

7 By storing your polish in the fridge you can make them last longer. Keeping it at a level temperature reduces the chances of it turning thick and gloopy, worth a try to save your favourite shade!

8 In the 1950s, red nails were considered 'promiscuous' and some churches even asked women to remove their nail polish on Sundays. This stigma stemmed from Victorian times, when nail polish was mostly worn by more promiscuous women and therefore considered sinful.

9 Darker nail polish shades are prone to chipping more easily. Due to the higher levels of pigment, they are naturally denser making them more likely to chip. Make them last a little longer by building up your colour in multiple thin coats.

10 Even your nails need a breather. Yes, you must part from your polish at least once a month and let nails be naked for a few days to keep them healthy and happy…your nails will love you for it.

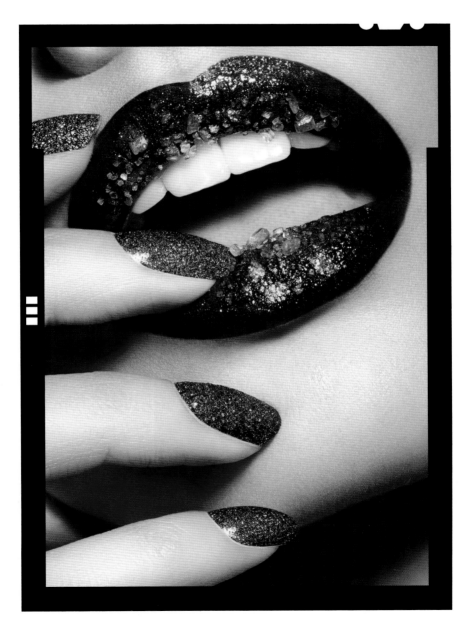

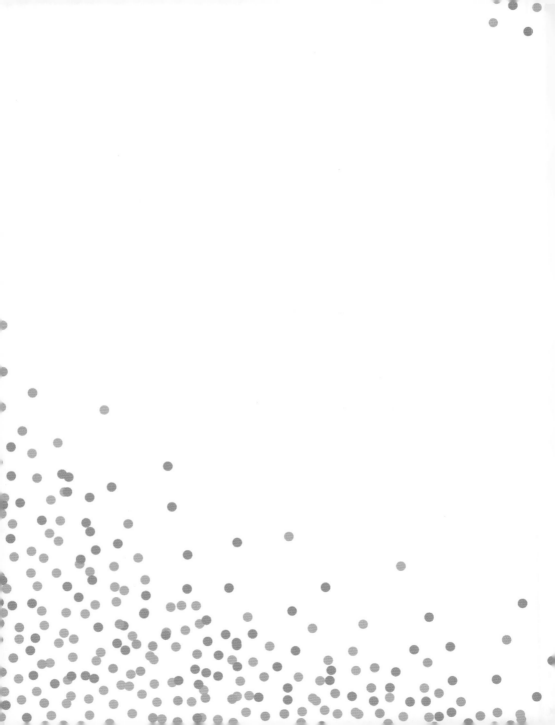

THE
STYLES

PILLARBOX PERFECTION

RED NAILS ARE ENDLESSLY CLASSIC AND WORK WITH ALMOST ANY AGE, OUTFIT, SKIN TONE OR EVENT. ONCE YOU HAVE THE PERFECT PAINT TECHNIQUE NAILED, THIS LOOK IS ONE YOU'LL RETURN TO TIME AND TIME AGAIN.

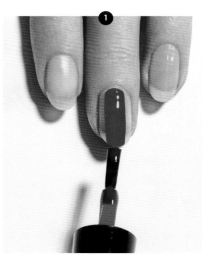
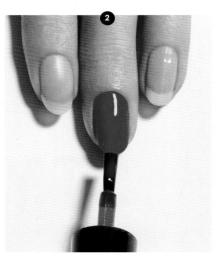

STEP BY STEP

1. Paint in three strokes – one stripe down the centre of the nail with one stripe either side. Repeat to add a second coat for a full coverage, opaque finish.

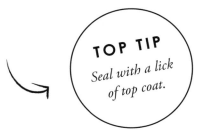

TOP TIP
Seal with a lick of top coat.

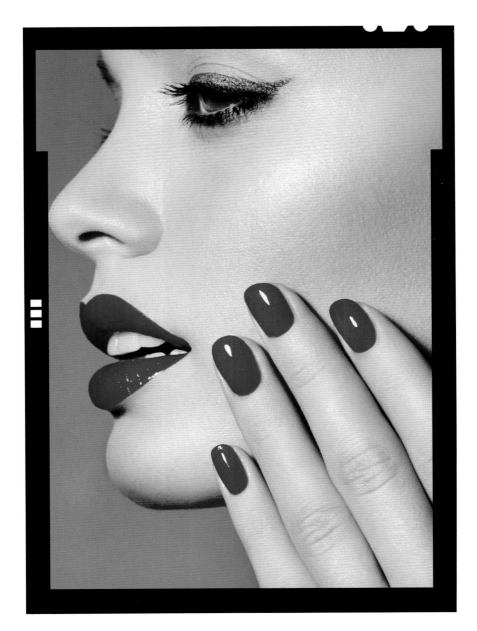

41

NEAT NEGATIVE SPACE

A SIMPLE YET CHIC WAY TO WEAR NEGATIVE SPACE NAILS
IS BY STICKING TO CLEAN LINES, FOR A CLASSIC NAIL
ENHANCING FINISH.

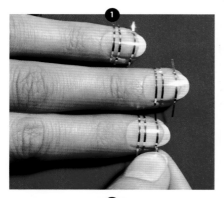

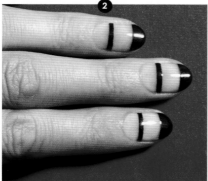

STEP BY STEP

1. Treat naked nails to a glossy base coat for added shine.

2. Lay two pieces of striping tape horizontally across the centre of each nail and one piece across the tip.

3. Using a skinny brush for neatness, fill in between the two pieces of striping tape on the centre of each nail and between the tape and the tip of the nail with a dark shade (we chose a deep blue).

TOP TIP
Wear with a lighter shade for a more subtle look.

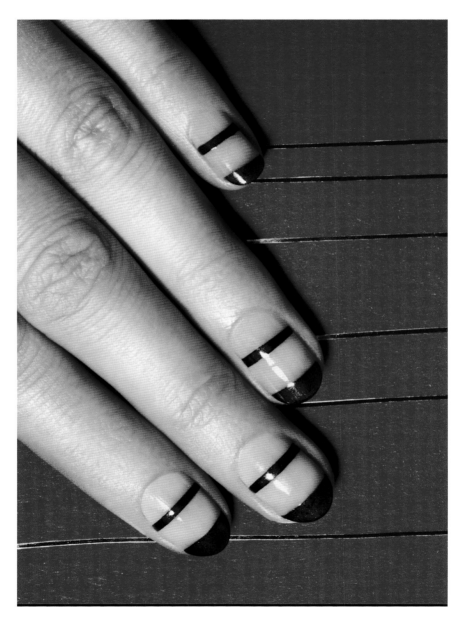

OVER THE MOON

THIS NAKED HALF-MOON MANI WAS WORN BY WOMEN IN THE 1930S AND HAS SINCE BECOME A RUNWAY FAVOURITE AND A GREAT WAY TO GIVE A CLASSIC RED MANICURE A VINTAGE TWIST.

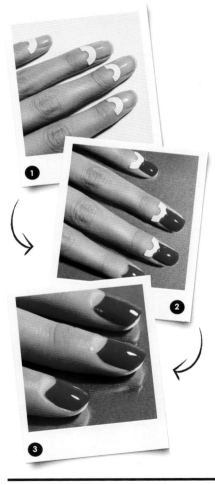

STEP BY STEP

1. Once your base coat is fully dry, stick hole punch reinforcement stickers to the base of each nail, positioned over the half moon.

2. Paint two coats of your chosen shade – use red for a classic vintage finish or wear with a bright shade for modern take on the look.

3. Once fully dry, peel away the stickers and add a glossy top coat over the whole of each nail.

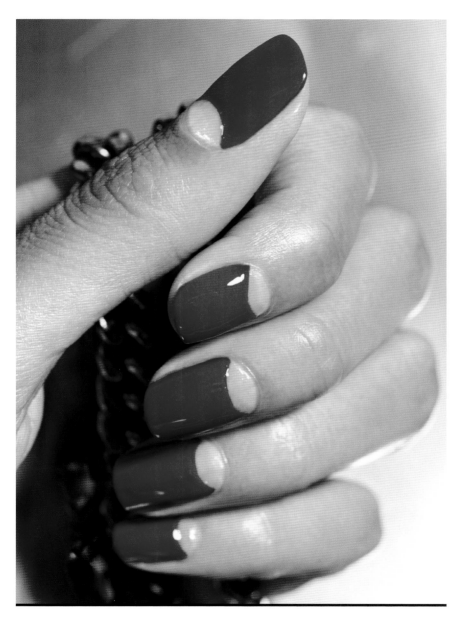

DOT TO DOT

OUTLINE AND ENHANCE THE SHAPE OF YOUR NAILS BY
ADDING SIMPLE SPOTTED DETAIL, TAKING YOUR MANI
FROM BORING TO BEAUTIFUL IN NO TIME.

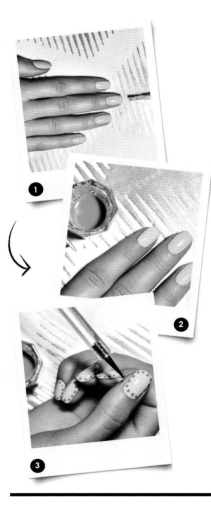

STEP BY STEP

1. Begin with a lighter base for maximum contrast – we painted nails in a pale pink.

2. Once your nails are dry, use a dotting tool and a darker shade, such as blue, to add drops of colour around the outer edges of the nails.

3. Leave to dry for about 20 minutes.

TOP TIP
Seal with a lick of top coat.

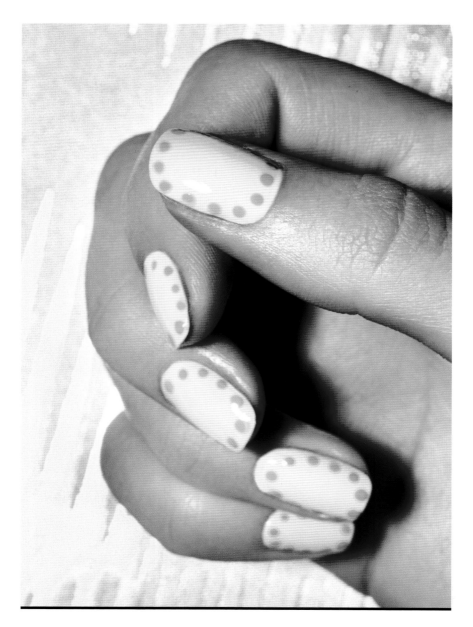

MOONBRIGHT

GIVE YOUR MANI A COLOUR-BLOCK TWIST BY ADDING
CONTRASTING COLOUR DETAILING – A SIMPLE WAY TO MAKE
YOUR FAVOURITE COLOUR POP. EASILY WEARABLE WITH
ANY SHADE OR TEXTURE. FIND YOUR FAVOURITE COLOUR
COMBINATIONS AND PAINT AWAY!

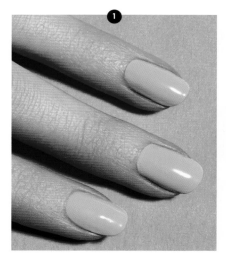
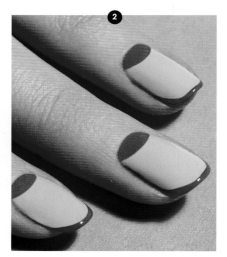

STEP BY STEP

1. Begin with a colourful base shade –
we painted nails in a pale peppermint
green.

2. With a striping brush, paint half-
moons and French tips in a contrasting
bright colour, such as bright pink.

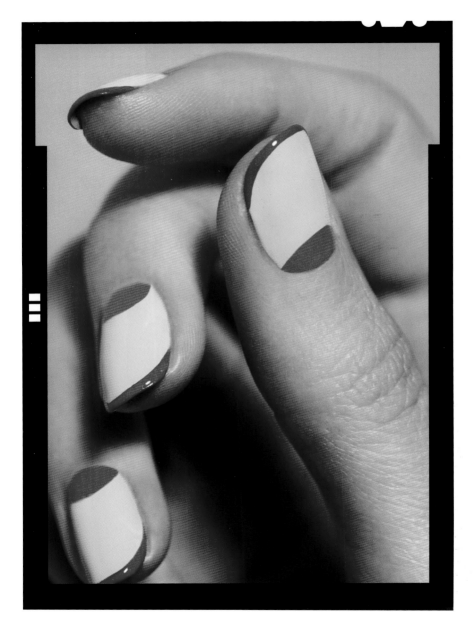

PASTEL POWER

WE'RE SO IN LOVE WITH PASTEL POLISH WE HAD TO FIND
A WAY TO WEAR THEM ALL AT ONCE! THIS SIMPLE SPONGING
TECHNIQUE GIVES A GORGEOUSLY SPECKLED FINISH.

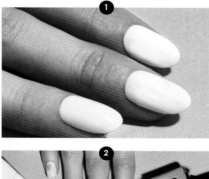

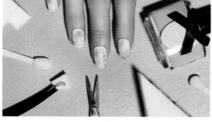

STEP BY STEP

1. Begin with a base of white polish for the perfect canvas.

2. To create the sponged look you can use a clean eye make-up applicator, or snip a small section of sponge and dab polish onto the nails using tweezers for a precision finish.

3. Dot a small amount of your chosen shade to the sponge and gently press to each nail.

4. Repeat in contrasting shades to layer colour – we used blue, pink, yellow, green and a darker purple.

TOP TIP
Seal with a lick
of top coat.

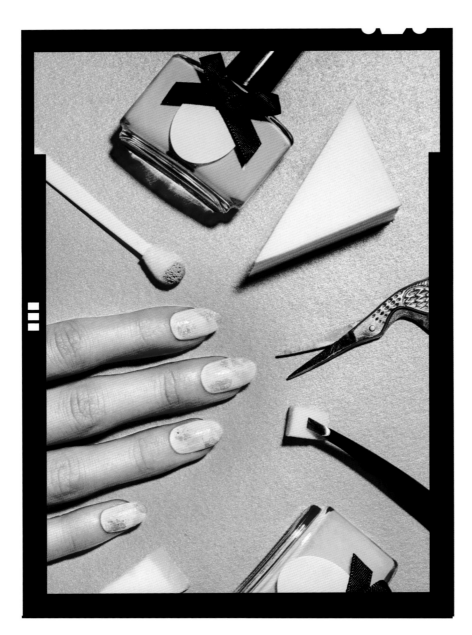

51

PEEK-A-BOO POLKA

INSPIRED BY LINGERIE TEXTILES, THIS CHEEKY SPOTTED STYLE
WILL ADD A FUN FINISH TO YOUR LOOK – WE CHOSE BLACK,
BUT YOU CAN RECREATE THIS STYLE IN ANY SHADE.

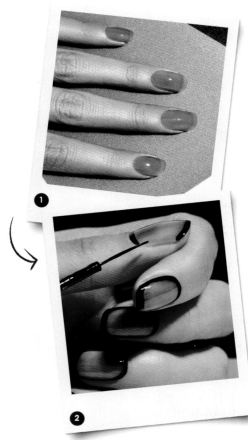

STEP BY STEP

1. Create a super sheer base by adding a few drops of black polish into some base coat and shake well to mix.

2. Paint the base on all nails and outline each nail with a dense black using a skinny nail art brush.

3. Use a dotting tool to place polka dots across the centre of the nail.

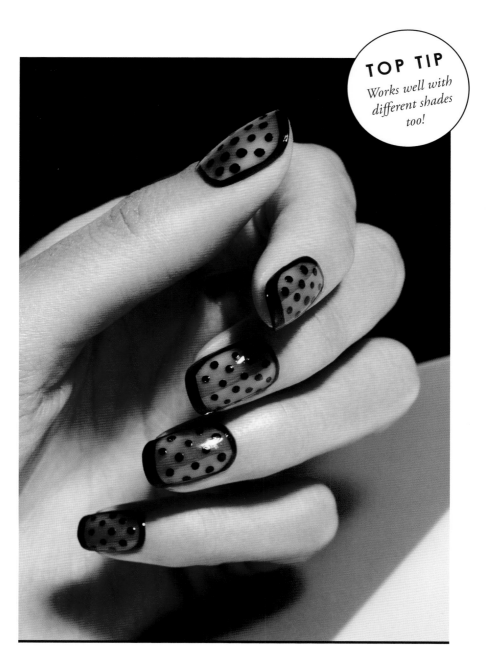

PAINTBOX PERFECTION

UNLEASH YOUR INNER ARTIST AND CREATE A MULTI-COLOURED
MASTERPIECE, USING THIS CLEVER BRUSH-STROKING TECHNIQUE.
NO STEADY HAND NEEDED, THIS LOOK IS MEANT TO BE MESSY
MAKING IT PERFECT FOR NAIL ART NEWBIES.

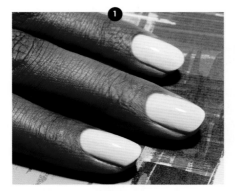

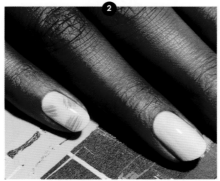

STEP BY STEP

1. Paint nails with a white base and
leave to dry for about 20 minutes.

2. Using a fan brush (see page 12), add
a tiny drop of polish to the bristles and
sweep the first colour onto the nails,
allowing them to dry fully.

3. Repeat this step to slowly build up
layers of colour, allowing the base shade
to peep out underneath.

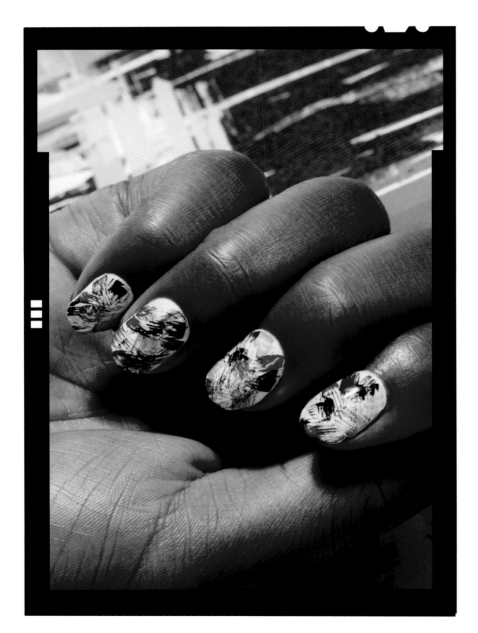

GALAXY NAILS

A FIRM FAVOURITE OF EVERY NAIL INSPIRATION PINTEREST
BOARD, THIS LOOK IS ALL ABOUT CLEVER COLOUR LAYERING
TO CREATE 'OUT-OF-THIS-WORLD' NAIL DESIGNS
(WE COULDN'T RESIST!)

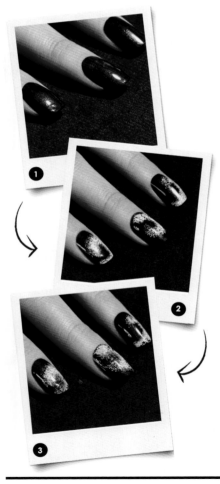

STEP BY STEP

1. Paint nails with a base coat of deep blue polish.

2. Add a small amount of white nail polish on a clean piece of sponge or an eye make-up applicator and gently dab onto the nails to create a flecked effect.

3. Paint with a top coat of sheer silver glitter polish for a galactic finish.

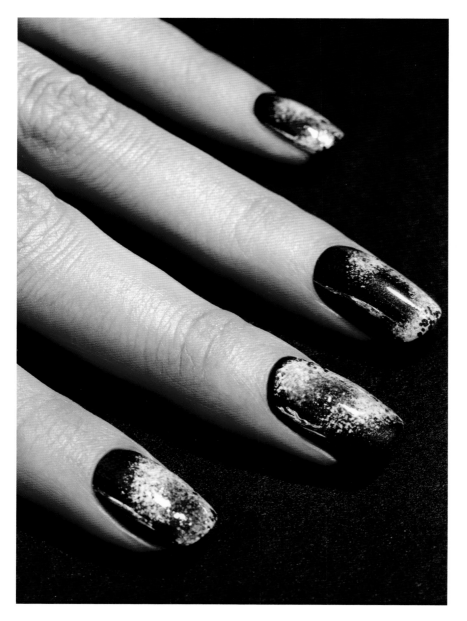

⤚✕⤛

CHARMED CHAIN

GIVE NAILS A LUXE TWIST BY CREATING DELICATE CHAINED DETAIL
DESIGNS – A GORGEOUS WAY TO ENHANCE YOUR JEWELLERY
AND TAKE YOUR MANI FROM DAY TO NIGHT IN AN INSTANT.

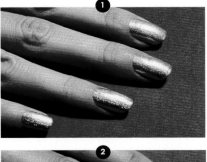

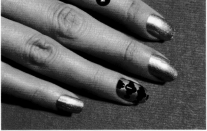

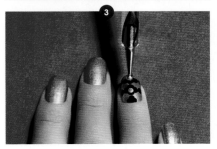

STEP BY STEP

1. Begin by painting nails with a metallic base shade – we've chosen a glimmering gold.

2. Use a dotting tool and a contrasting colour, such as glossy black, to create an intricate chain pattern over the nail on your ring finger. Leave to dry for about 20 minutes.

3. Clean the dotting tool and fill in the pattern using the base shade but leaving a contrasting outline to create a chain-like effect.

4. Wear as an accent nail on your ring finger or repeat on all ten nails for an all-out look.

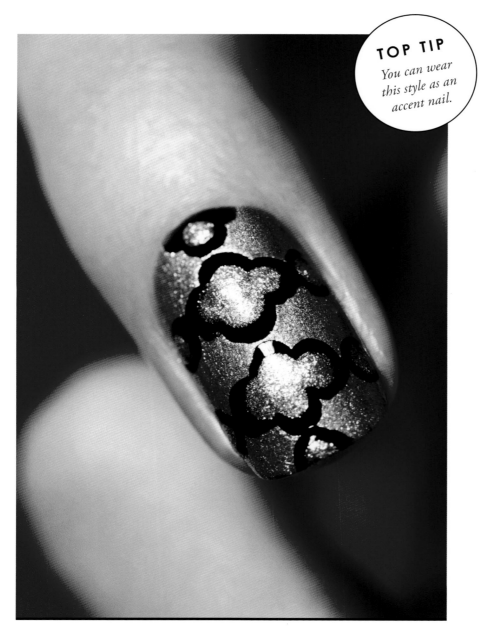

TOP TIP
*You can wear
this style as an
accent nail.*

GEOMETRIC FRENCH TIPS

ADD A FLASH OF COLOUR TO YOUR NAIL TIPS BY CREATING
THESE SUPER PRETTY FRENCH TIPS WITH A GEOMETRIC TWIST. IF
YOU DON'T HAVE CONTRASTING SHADES, CHOOSE A DARKER
SHADE AND ADD A DROP OF WHITE POLISH TO MIX YOUR OWN
CONTRASTING LIGHTER SHADE.

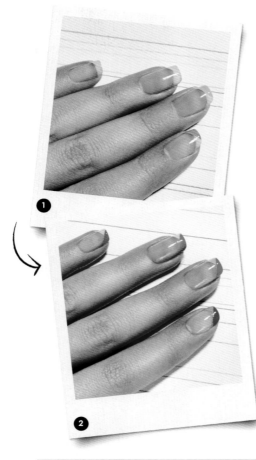

STEP BY STEP

1. Treat naked nails to a glossy base coat for added shine.

2. With a striping brush, paint a diagonal stipe of colour to the bottom corner of each nail tip. You can use the same colour for each nail or choose a range of shades as we did.

3. Once dry, paint a darker tone of the same shade in the other corner to complete the look.

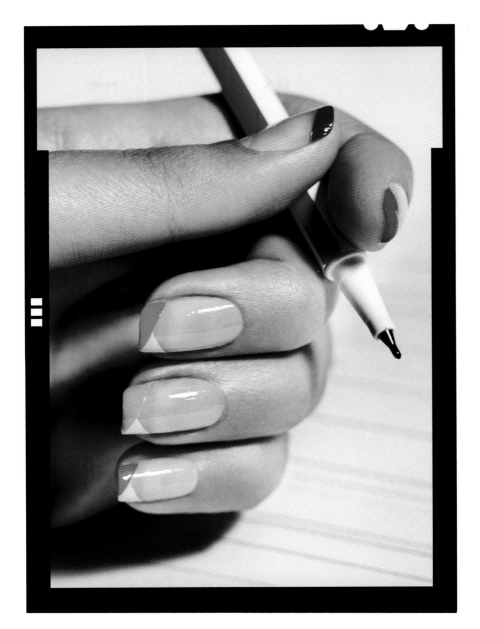

⤝⤞

NEON COLOUR CLASH

PERFECT FOR GIVING TANNED HANDS A SUMMERY STATEMENT, THIS
TRIANGL BIKINI-INSPIRED NAIL ART IS NOT ONLY SERIOUSLY FUN BUT
A FRESH WAY TO WEAR NEON POLISH.

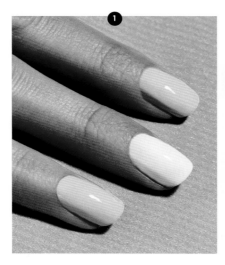

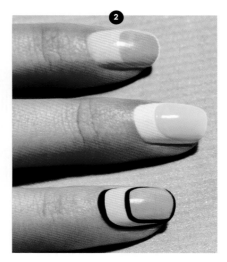

STEP BY STEP

1. Begin by painting alternating shades of white and almost white on nails.

2. Once dry, paint two neon shades over three-quarters of each nail, leaving a contrasting piece of base shade peeking through.

3. Outline the full nail and contrasting nude section using black polish on a skinny brush to make the shades pop.

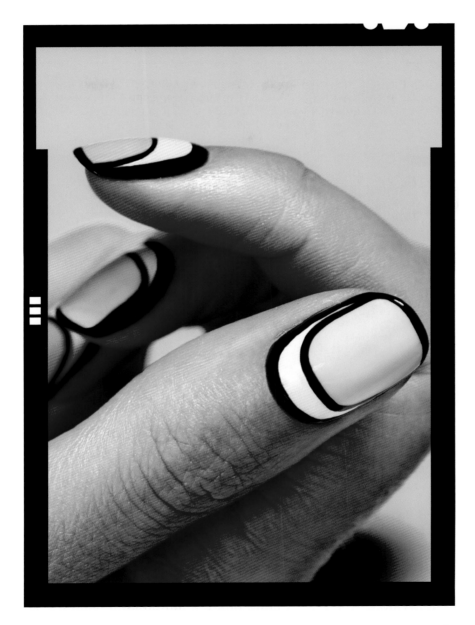

IN THE NUDE

GIVE NUDE A FASHIONABLE TWIST, BY LAYERING SEVERAL
SHADES IN THIS CLEVER CONTOURED SHAPE, MAKING NAILS
LOOK LONGER AND MORE SLENDER. THIS ELONGATING TRICK
IS A GREAT TECHNIQUE TO MASTER.

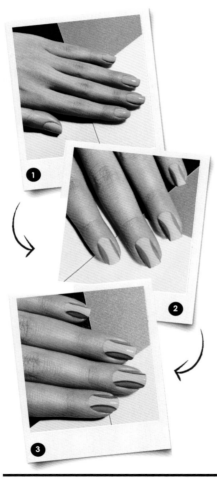

STEP BY STEP

1. Begin by painting nails with a base of
a light nude shade.

2. Once dry, paint curved lines from
the base to the tip on both sides of each
nail using a slightly darker shade and a
skinny brush. Fill in each side and leave
to dry for about 20 minutes.

3. Finally, finish with a skinny line
between the centre and curved blocks
on each side of the nail in an even
darker shade of nude.

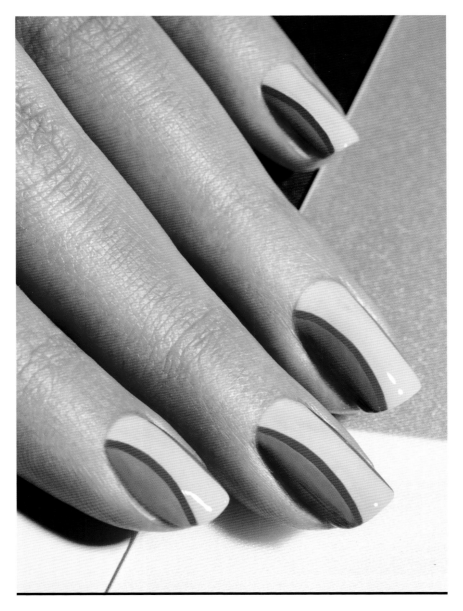

⤝⤞

SPOT ON

LEOPARD SPOTS ARE ALWAYS STYLISH. WE'VE GIVEN OURS
A GIRLY TWIST BY USING A LILAC BASED COLOUR PALETTE –
MIX UP YOUR SHADE COMBOS TO CREATE A UNIQUE FINISH.

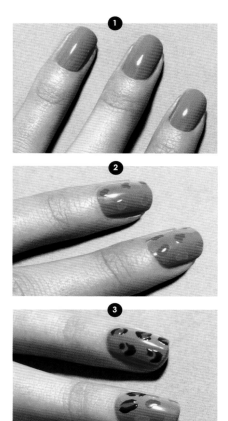

STEP BY STEP

1. Paint nails in your selected base shade and allow to dry fully.

2. Using a dotting tool, scatter curved splodges in a darker contrasting shade over the nails and allow to dry.

3. Using a clean dotting tool, outline half of each dot with black to give it a leopard print look. You can also add a few small black dots to the nails too.

TOP TIP
Seal with a lick of top coat.

66

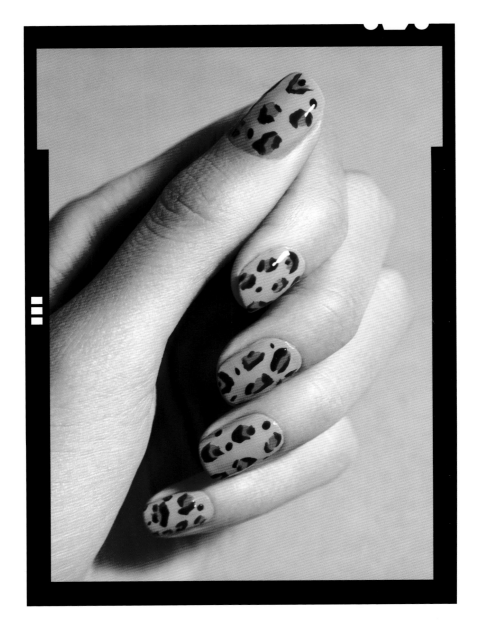

WATER MARBLING

WATER MARBLING CAN BE TRICKY TO MASTER, BUT IT'S
A PERFECT WAY TO ADD MULTIPLE LAYERS OF COLOUR
FOR A TOTALLY UNIQUE NAIL LOOK.

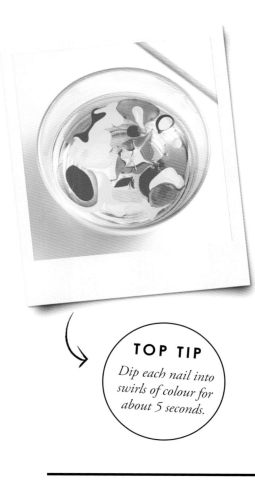

STEP BY STEP

1. Prepare a cup of water – marbling won't work in cold water as it hardens the polish instantly, so set aside for a few hours until room temperature.

2. Select the shades you'd like to marble with and add one drop of each colour to the water. Repeat as often as you wish – the more drops you add, the closer the colours will sit next to each other.

3. Using an orange wood stick, draw lines through the polish to pull the colours together and create a rippled 'marble' effect.

4. Prep the nails with a layer of base coat and add liquid nail tape or masking tape around the cuticle and fingertip to minimise mess. Dip each nail into the swirl of colour and hold for about 5 seconds.

5. Remove fingers and clean away excess paint by peeling away the liquid nail tape from the edge of nails or removing masking tape. Complete your swirled polish with a glossy top coat.

TOP TIP

Dip each nail into swirls of colour for about 5 seconds.

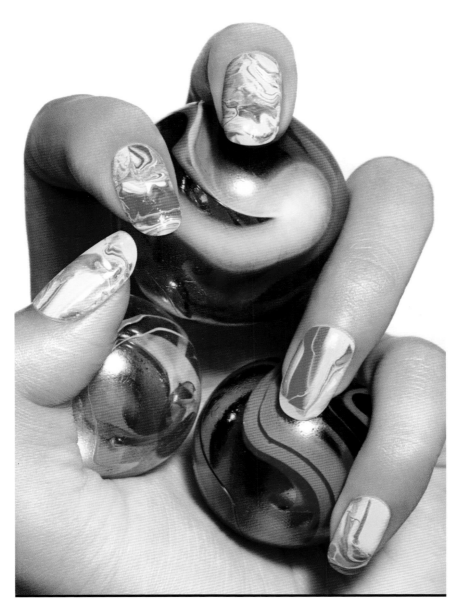

MONOCHROME

BLACK AND WHITE IS THE NEW BLACK – MONOCHROME
IS FOREVER A FASHION STAPLE AND MIXING THIS CLASSIC
SHADE COMBO IN CLEAN GEOMETRIC LINES IS A SIMPLE WAY
TO CREATE A STRIKING NAIL LOOK.

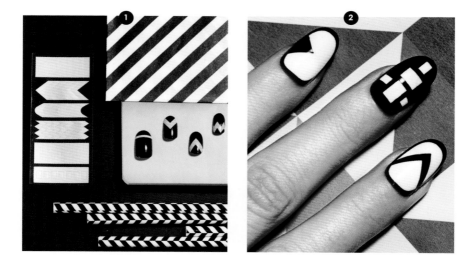

STEP BY STEP

1. Paint nails with a base shade of white and allow to dry completely.

2. Using pattern guides, lay your chosen cut out onto each nail.

3. Paint a coat of black polish over the white base and pattern guides and allow to dry.

4. Peel away the pattern guides to reveal your monochrome look. Add a slick of top coat for extra gloss.

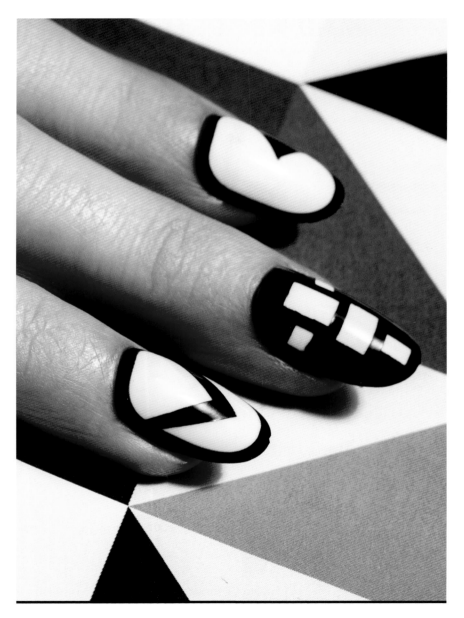

MAD ABOUT MATTE

MIX UP YOUR MATTE MANI BY ADDING SERIOUSLY SHINY STYLING
DETAILS – SUPER SIMPLE YET EFFORTLESSLY EFFECTIVE.

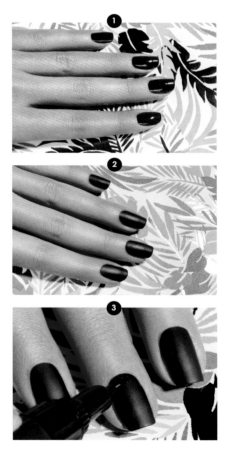

STEP BY STEP

1. Begin by painting the nails with a base of your chosen shade.

2. Once dry, add a matte top coat to transform the finish from shiny to matte.

3. Using a nail art pen or skinny dotting tool, add a traingular dotted pattern to each nail using the glossy base colour.

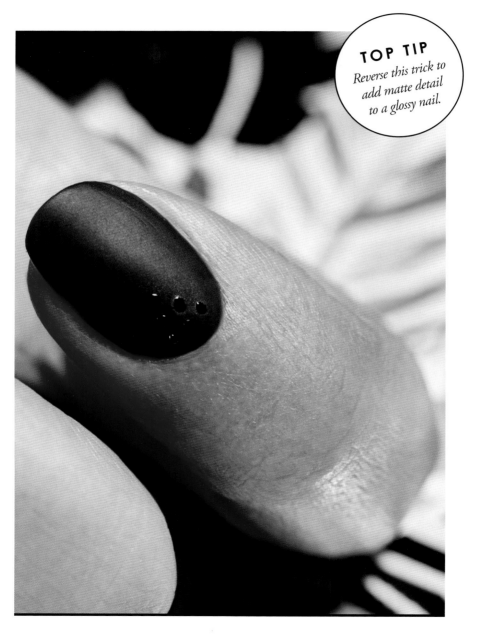

FLOATING MANI

NAIL THE MONOCHROME NAIL TREND BY CREATING A
FLOATING MANICURE – MUCH LOVED BY BACKSTAGE NAIL
TECHNICIANS AND BLOGGERS ALIKE, THIS STRIKING LOOK
IS SURPRISINGLY SIMPLE TO ACHIEVE.

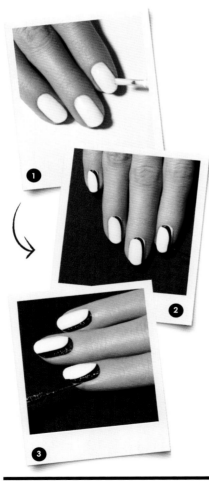

STEP BY STEP

1. Start by painting nails with a white base coat and leave to dry.

2. Paint a solid black curved stripe over the cuticle and down the left edge of the nail in black.

3. Fill the rest of the edge with dense black glitter.

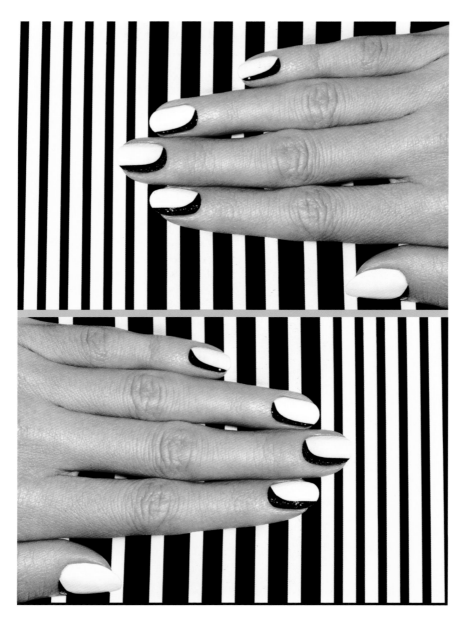

TRIANGULAR TRICKS

TRANSFORM A CLASSIC NUDE BASE BY ADDING A TWIST OF
GLITTER. USE STRIPING TAPE TO PAINT THE PERFECT TRIANGLE.

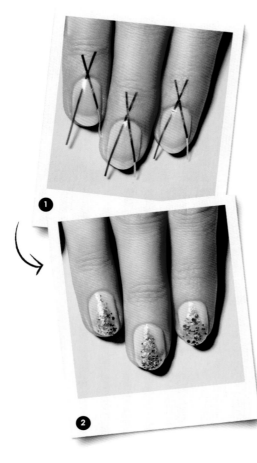

STEP BY STEP

1. Begin by painting nails with a nude polish and leave to dry completely.

2. Add striping tape from the centre of the cuticles down to the corner of the nails and repeat on the opposite side to create a symmetrical triangle.

3. Paint inside the striping tape with a glitter polish and leave to dry for about 20 minutes. Peel away the tape to reveal geometric glitter triangles.

TOP TIP
Seal with a lick
of top coat.

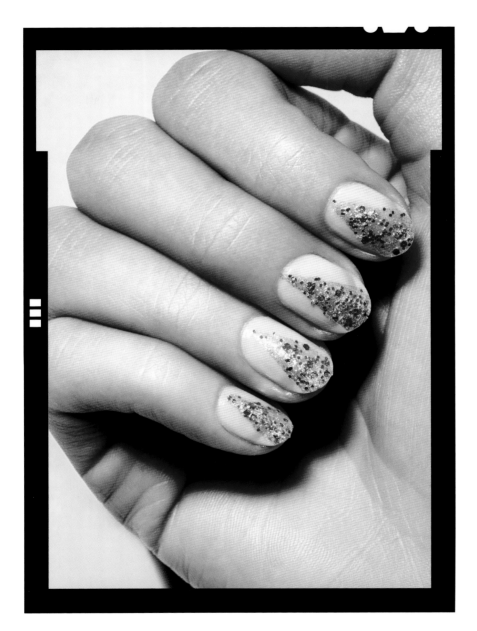

GLITTER GRADIENT

THIS IS THE PERFECT WAY TO TRANSFORM A CLASSIC DAYTIME LOOK INTO A PARTY READY FINISH, AND IS ALSO A GREAT WAY TO CONCEAL ANY NAIL CHIPPING.

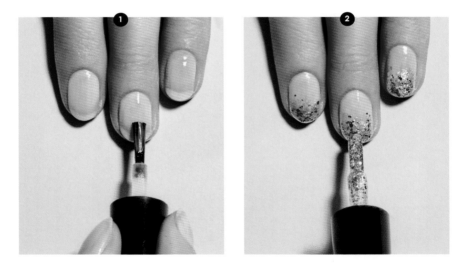

STEP BY STEP

1. Paint a nude base for a nail-enhancing look.

2. Dab gold glitter onto nail tips and extend up to middle of the nail, using a matching glitter polish.

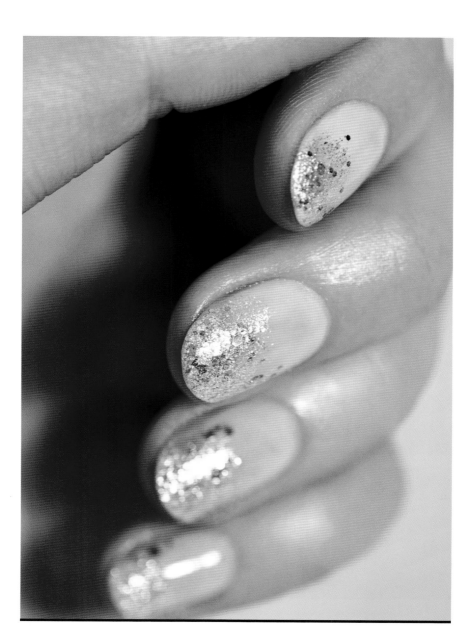

GLITTER GLAMOUR

THIS SUPER SIMPLE TECHNIQUE IS PERFECT FOR QUICKLY
ADDING A GLAMOROUS TWIST TO ANY PAINT JOB.

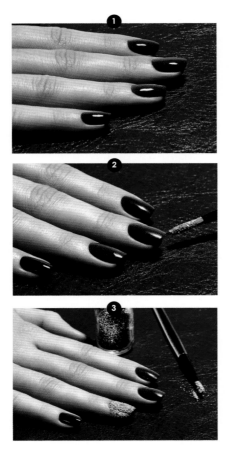

STEP BY STEP

1. Paint a base colour of your choice – we chose a deep khaki green.

2. Using loose glitter, gently tap over the wet polish on the accent nail using a soft flat brush.

3. Sweep away excess glitter when you are done.

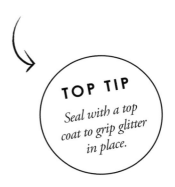

TOP TIP

Seal with a top coat to grip glitter in place.

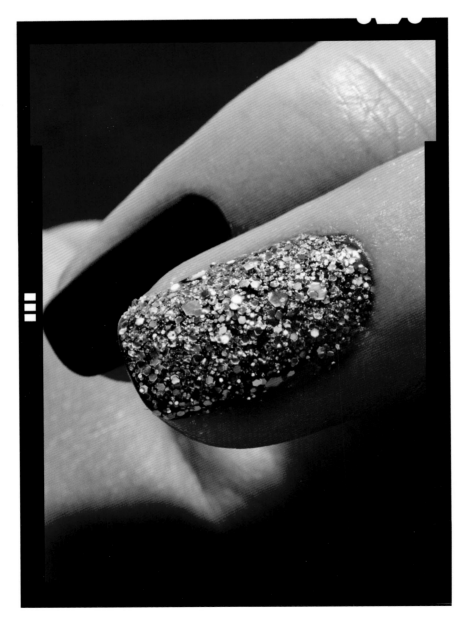

BEACH-READY OMBRE

INSPIRED BY SUNSET OMBRÉ SKIES, THIS DIP-DYED FINISH
IS PERFECT WHEN PAIRED WITH A BIKINI. ADD A GLITTER TOP
COAT TO NOT ONLY GIVE A SPARKLING PARTY FINISH,
BUT TO LOCK IN YOUR LOOK FOR LONGER.

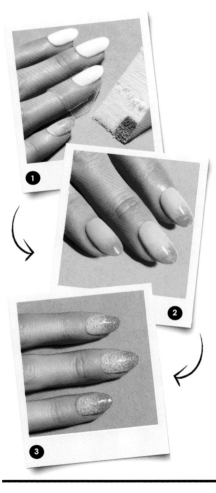

STEP BY STEP

1. Begin by painting nails with a base coat of white polish.

2. Drop two shades of the same colour on to a sponge, allowing them to bleed slightly into each other.

3. Gently dab the colour onto the nails and leave to dry completely.

4. Complete with a sheer glittering top coat if desired.

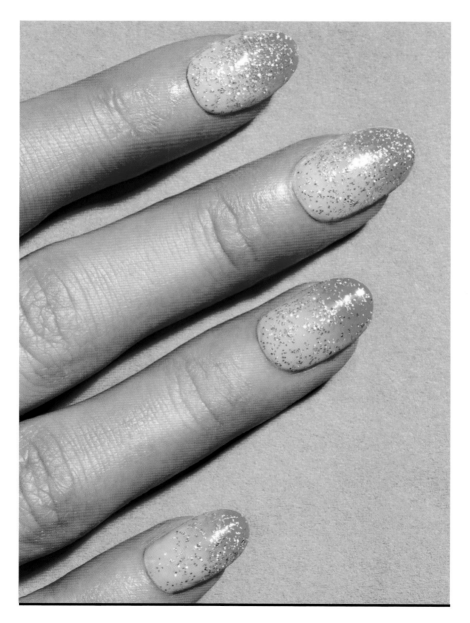

SWEET SHOP SPOTS

THIS IS THE LAZY GIRL'S WAY TO ACHIEVE A NAIL ART
FINISH BY USING DENSE GLITTER POLISH TO GIVE A SUGARY-
SWEET LOOK. THE ADDED COLOURFUL FRENCH TIP
IS A GREAT WAY TO ENHANCE NAIL SHAPE.

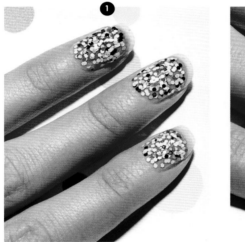
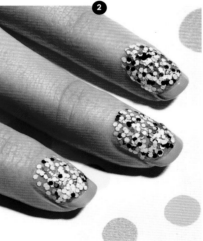

STEP BY STEP

1. Paint three coats of dense, multi-coloured glitter onto the nails, skipping the tips, for a full coverage look.

2. Complete the look by painting a contrasting colourful French tip to match your glitter shade using a skinny brush.

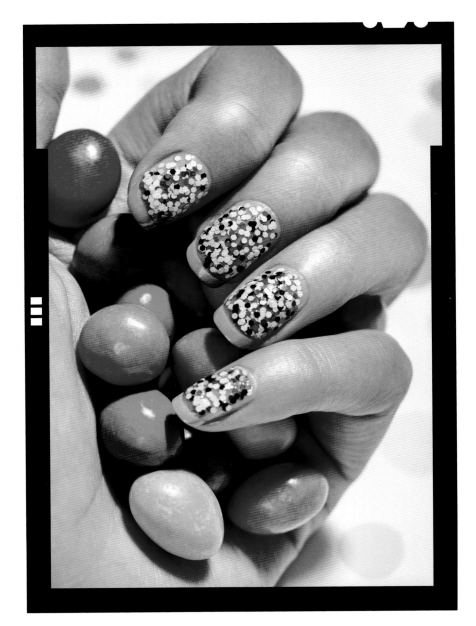

CRUSHED VELVET

THE USE OF THIS DECADENT TEXTURE GIVES NAILS A RUNWAY INSPIRED LOOK AT THE SPRINKLE OF A VELVET SHAKER – MADE FAMOUS BY CIATÉ IN 2012, THIS FUZZY FASHION-FORWARD FINISH IS A FUN WAY TO EXPERIMENT WITH NAIL ART.

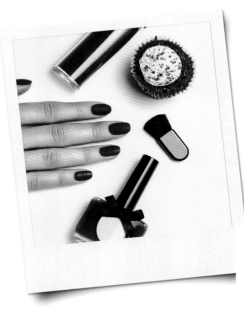

STEP BY STEP

1. Begin by painting the nails with a base of block colour to match the velvet powder.

2. While nails are wet, shake a generous coating of velvet powder over each nail for a fuzzy finish. Leave to dry completely.

3. Be sure to avoid staining the velvet finish when touching liquids or oils.

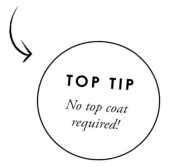

TOP TIP

No top coat required!

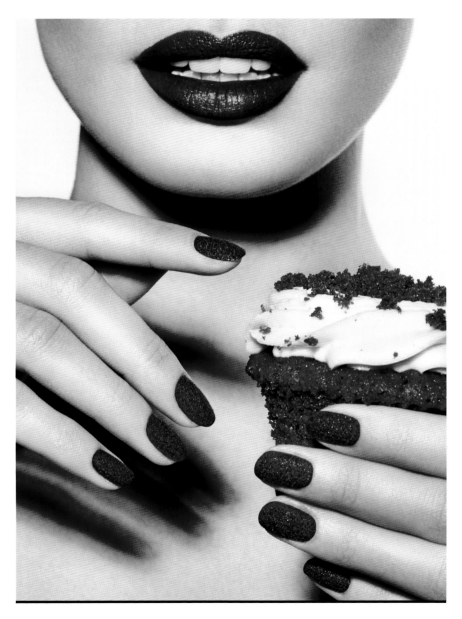

SIMPLE STUDS

STUDS DON'T ALWAYS MEAN GRUNGE GOTHIC GLAMOUR –
ACHIEVE AN UNDERSTATED LOOK WITH THIS SIMPLE TECHNIQUE,
THE PERFECT WAY TO ENHANCE A RICH POLISH COLOUR.

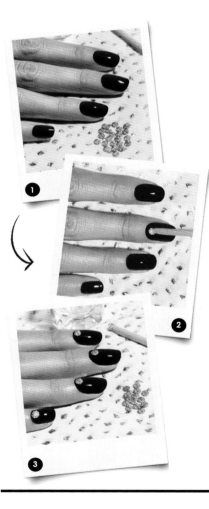

STEP BY STEP

1. Paint nails with a base coat of deep red polish.

2. Using an orange wood stick, add a drop of nail glue to the back of each embellishment and place at the base of each nail. Leave to dry for about 20 minutes.

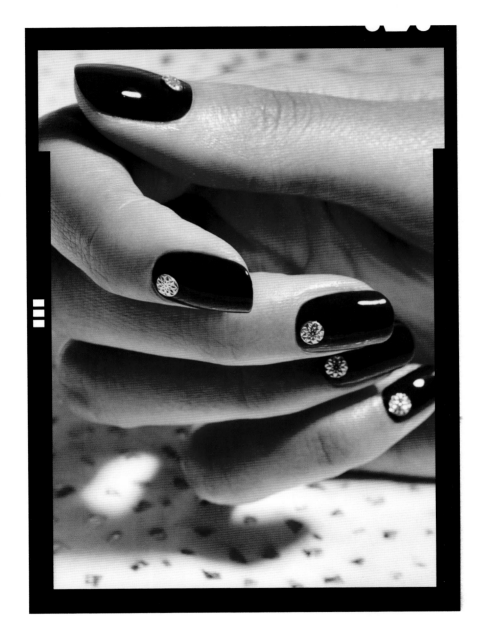

NEGATIVE SPACE STUDS

AMP UP YOUR STUDDED LOOK BY GIVING IT A NEGATIVE SPACE
TWIST. WE LOVE THE NATURAL NAIL PEEKING OUT UNDERNEATH
TO BALANCE THE GOLD STUDS GIVING A MODERN FINISH.

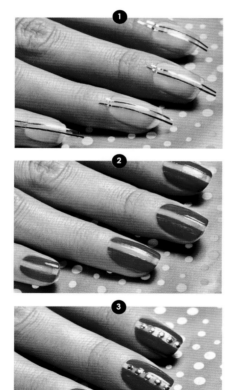

STEP BY STEP

1. To create the negative space, divide along the centre of the nail using two pieces of striping tape.

2. Carefully paint either side of each nail using a dense crème colour, such as a strong red.

3. When completely dry, finish the look by carefully placing stud embellishments along the centre of the nail using an orange wood stick and a dot of base coat.

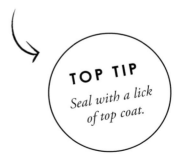

TOP TIP
Seal with a lick
of top coat.

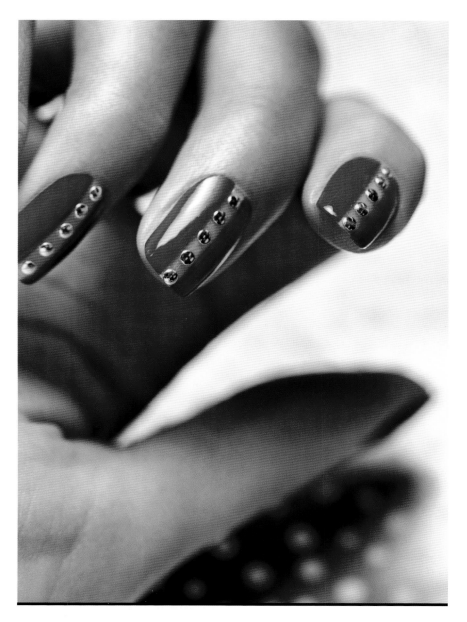

CHAMPAGNE AND CAVIAR

THIS CULT CLASSIC HELPED TO PUT CIATÉ ON THE BEAUTY MAP
IN 2012 WHEN I USED IT ON A PHOTOSHOOT
– THE REST IS HISTORY!

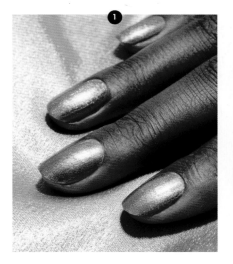

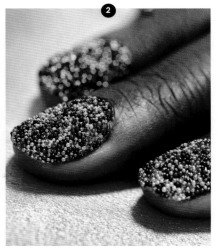

STEP BY STEP

1. Paint a base colour of your choice – we went for a glittering champagne gold. Prepare the nail for caviar pearls by painting another heavier coat of polish and while still wet sprinkle the beads onto the nail. Gently pat the beads into the polish to secure them in place.

2. This can't be worn with a coat of top coat, but you can seal in the caviar pearls with a thin sweep of top coat across the very tip of each nail. Allow to set for 20–30 minutes to avoid any dropping pearls.

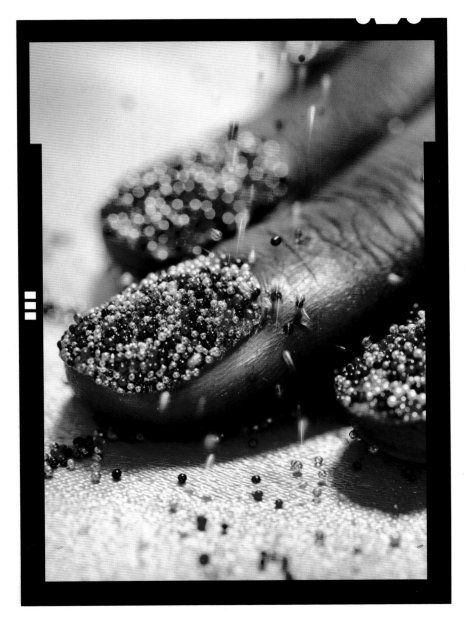

GET PERSONAL

MAKE YOUR MANI TRULY YOUR OWN BY ADDING A
PERSONAL TWIST. WE LOVE STAMPED OUT INITIALS FOR A
MONOGRAMMED MANI, OR SPELL OUT YOUR OWN
MESSAGE WHATEVER THE OCCASION!

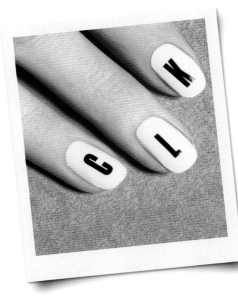

STEP BY STEP

1. Start by painting nails with a white base and allow to dry completely.

2. Cut out your selected letter, wet the reverse of the transfer then press and hold onto the nail for 10–15 seconds.

3. Gently peel away the backing to reveal your transfer – always seal with a slick of top coat.

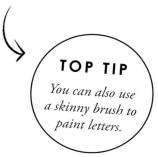

TOP TIP

You can also use a skinny brush to paint letters.

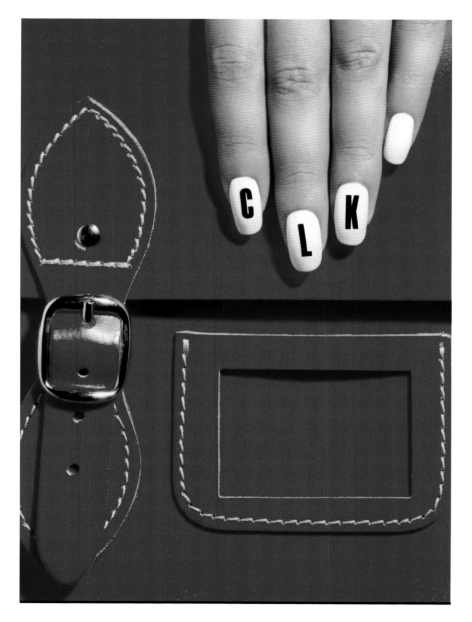

✄

COLOURFOIL

ADD FOILING TO NAILS FOR OUT-OF-THIS-WORLD TEXTURE AND
SHINE – THE PERFECT WAY TO DRESS UP A SIMPLE MANI.

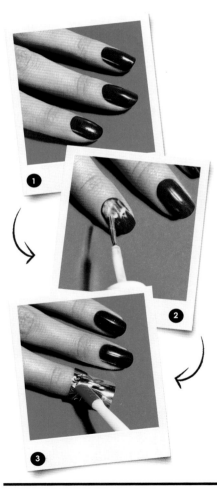

STEP BY STEP

1. Begin by painting nails with a base coat of your favourite shade – choose a colour that complements the foil.

2. Once fully dry, paint a coat of glue onto the nails where you want the foil to be placed.

3. When the glue is slightly tacky to touch, place the foil shiny side up and press to the nail. Peel away to reveal your shimmering design.

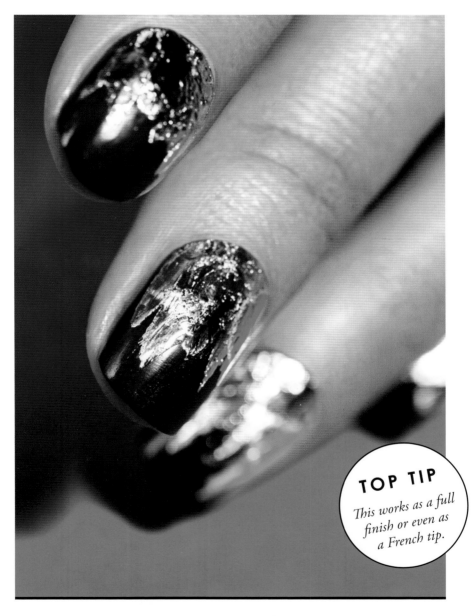

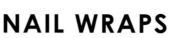

NAIL WRAPS

THIS IS THE LAZY GIRL'S WAY TO CREATE INCREDIBLY
INTRICATE DESIGNS IN AN INSTANT.

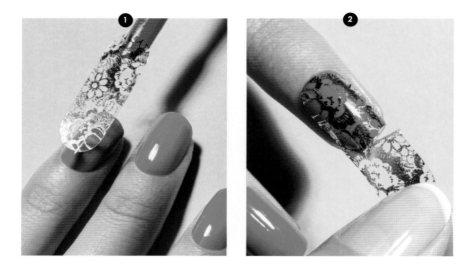

STEP BY STEP

1. Nail wraps come in an endless variety of patterns and textures, our favourites are sheer designs that allow the base shade of polish to peep through. Paint your nails in a solid base colour.

2. Simply select a wrap that best fits your nail size and press over the nail (when the polish is completely dry). Trim away excess wrap using nail scissors and file the edge of the nail for a clean finish.

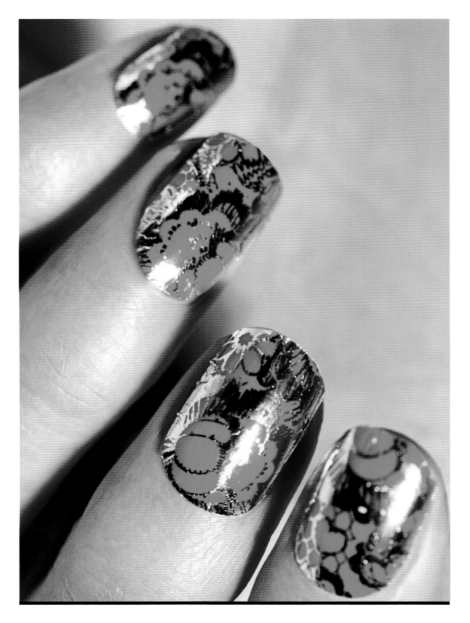

EXPERIMENT WITH TOP COATS

THE SIMPLEST WAY TO TRANSFORM YOUR NAIL POLISH
COLLECTION IS BY PLAYING WITH TEXTURES USING A MATTE TOP
COAT TO CREATE A FASHION-FORWARD, TEXTURED TWIST TO
YOUR MANICURE.

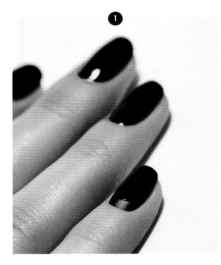

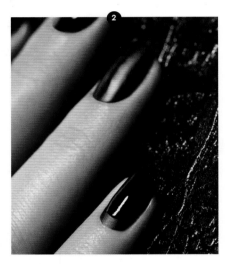

STEP BY STEP

1. Play with contrasting textures using a matte top coat to give nails a subtle nail art twist. Paint nails in a shiny base colour.

2. Paint full accent nails or add a subtle matte French tip with a matte top coat to give nails an eye-catching finish.

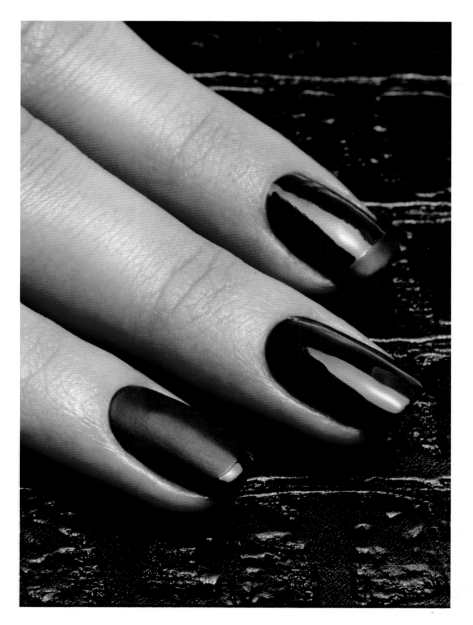

LAYERING POLISH SHADES

COLOURBLOCKING IS FOREVER IN FAVOUR AND GEOMETRIC
PATTERNS ARE THE BEST WAY TO WEAR THIS TREND ON YOUR
NAILS. THIS MODERN MONDRIAN-INSPIRED DESIGN IS A GREAT
WAY TO LOAD UP YOUR LOOK WITH COLOUR.

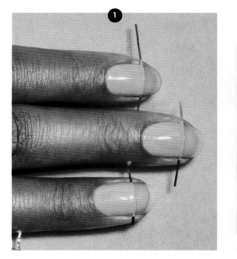 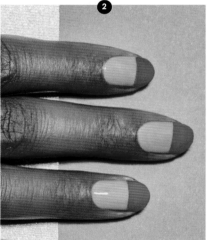

STEP BY STEP

1. Add striping tape horizontally across the centre line of the nail.

2. Paint nails in contrasting shades in the top and bottom section.

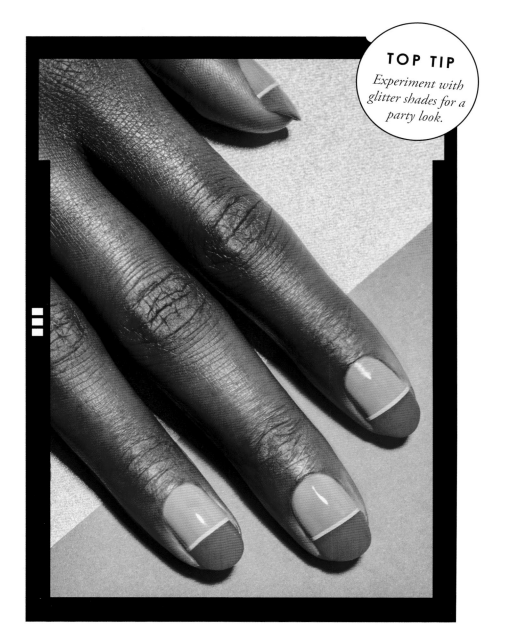

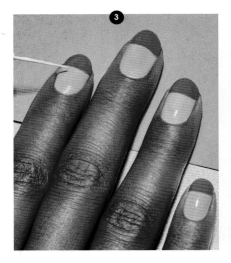

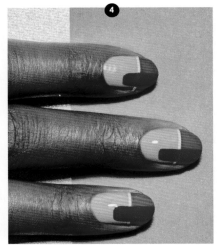

3. Once fully dry, peel away the tape and draw a skinny white line horizontally across the nail.

4. Using a skinny brush, paint a box of colour vertically to cover a quarter of the nail in a contrasting shade.

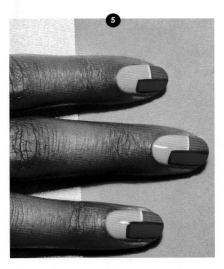

5. Complete the look by adding an outline to the box in another contrasting colour.

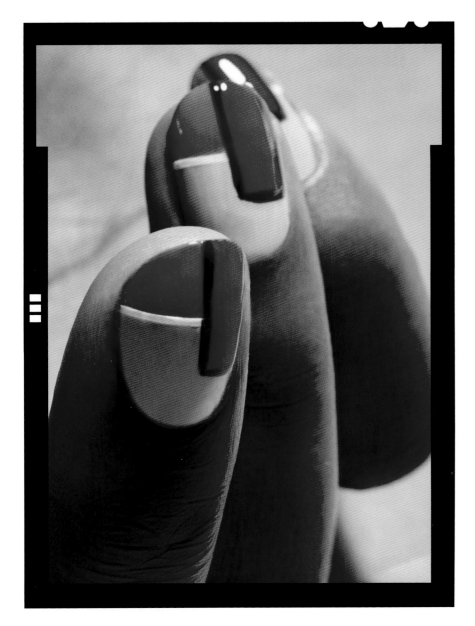

JEWELLED

FOR AN ALL-OUT EMBELLISHED LOOK, ENCRUST NAILS IN SPARKLING JEWELS TO GIVE THEM SERIOUS STAND-OUT APPEAL. PAIRED WITH A RICH BASE SHADE, THIS IS A GREAT WAY TO GIVE YOUR MANI A DECADENT FINISH.

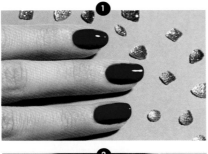

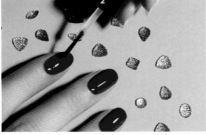

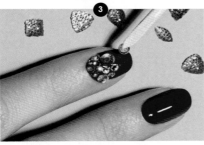

STEP BY STEP

1. Paint your nails in a shade that most complements your selection of stones – rich jewelled tones usually work best.

2. Once fully dry, paint the nail with a top coat and lay each stone onto the wet nail to set in place using an orange wood stick.

3. Wear on your ring finger or on all nails for a full-on finish.

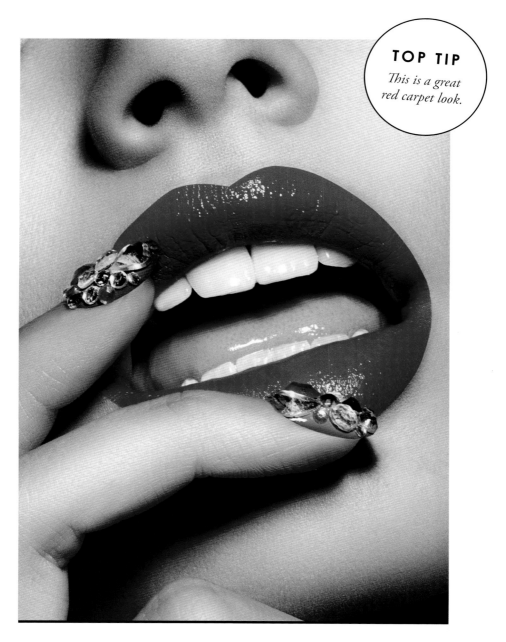

GLOBAL NAIL STYLES

LOOKING AT NAIL STYLING ON AN INTERNATIONAL LEVEL
IS A GREAT WAY OF GETTING INSPIRATION FOR DIFFERENT NAIL
LOOKS AND TECHNIQUES. FROM ANCIENT TRADITIONS TO THE
LATEST CUTTING EDGE INNOVATIONS, I CAN'T HELP BUT BE
FASCINATED BY GLOBAL INFLUENCES.

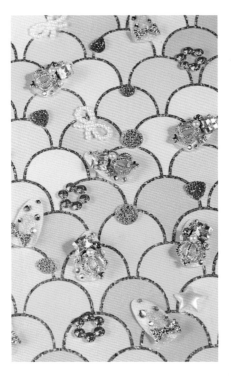

Key countries have their very own distinguishable nail styling, most predominantly in Japan where well-trained 'nailists' have become leaders in innovative nail designs. The nail art scene in Japan is massive with magazines, accessories and entire expos devoted to blinged-out nails. Intricate 3D designs are most iconic, the more embellishment the better!

Temporary cuticle tattoos became fashionable a couple of years ago, and are a great way to extend designs across the fingertips. Traditionally, Maori tribes in New Zealand have decorated their hands and bodies with intricate designs in a practice which dates back thousands of years. The technique is done without a modern tattoo needle using a chisel, ink pigment and a mallet. We'd much rather stick to temporary tats!

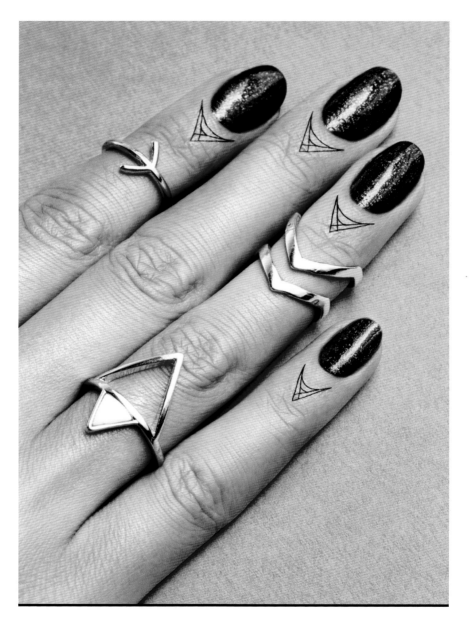

STYLE MENU

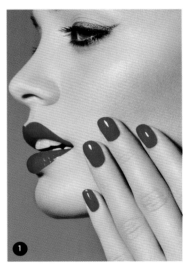

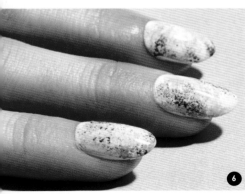

1 Pillarbox Perfection

2 Neat Negative Space

3 Over the Moon

4 Dot to Dot

5 Moonbright

6 Pastel Power

7 Peek-a-boo Polka

8 Paintbox Perfection

9 Galaxy Nails

10 Charmed Chain

11 Geometric French Tips

12 Neon Colour Clash

13 In the Nude

14 Spot On

15 Water Marbling

16 Monochrome

17 Mad about Matte

18 Floating Mani

19 Triangular Tricks

20 Glitter Gradient

21 Glitter Glamour

22 Beach-ready Ombre

23 Sweet Shop Spots

24 Crushed Velvet

25 Simple Studs

26 Negative Space Studs

27 Champagne and Caviar

28 Get Personal

29 Colourfoil

30 Nail Wraps

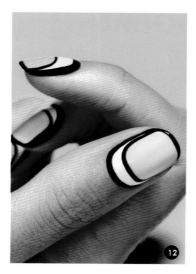

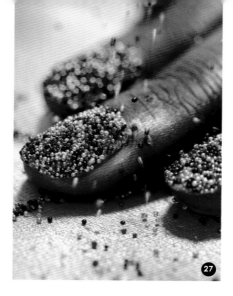

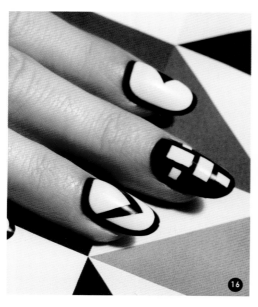

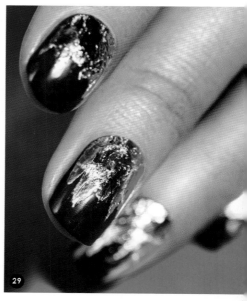

ACKNOWLEDGEMENTS

The love of a family is life's greatest blessing, so I must start by thanking my grandmother, Marie. You started my passion for fashion and inspired my love of accessories and shoes from a young age – I always remember staring up at your huge closet filled with shoe boxes in awe! You always looked sophisticated, glamorous and perfectly polished.

Thank you to my wonderful mother, Suzy, through your positive mantras, spiritual guidance and child-like wonderment, you have helped me manage stress and negative situations throughout my life and career.

My angel daughter, Gracie, thank you for inspiring me every day, through arts and crafts time, exploring your incredible imagination and your infectious laughter and smile…. Watching you grow into the stunning young lady you are becoming fills my heart full of joy.

A massive thank you to my wonderful best friend and PR guru for so many years, Sally Anne. Being on this journey with my best friend by my side is magical and a dream come true.

Thank you to all my wonderful friends and family for your patience and loyalty over the years; our friendship and love is still so strong even when we must spend months apart whilst juggling families and careers.

I would like to thank my wonderful team of incredibly passionate, talented individuals. Without you, none of this would have been possible. A special thank you to my uber creative dream team, Sophie Huddy and Hannah Griffiths, for your creativity and energy in creating our book and in all that you do. A huge thanks to Rebecca Jade Wilson, your craft continues to blow my mind… and Claire Harrison for your spectacular art behind the lens. Huge love to the ever beautiful chameleon that is Stacey Hannant, our cover star, and the fabulous hands of Brittany, Eleanor, Gemma, Kate, Krystle, Lauren, Leanne, Samira and Vicky who helped to create this book. You are all beautiful inside and out.

Thank you to Kyle Cathie, Vicky Orchard and the Kyle Books team – without you this project would have remained a dream – your guidance and drive has truly captured the talent and passion of the Ciaté team and we can't wait to share it with the world!

And finally, a gigantic thank you to you, the reader, for buying our book and sharing our passion for beauty – at Ciaté we count every fan as a best friend and we wouldn't be here without you. We can't wait to share our next chapter with you!